KEEP WEIGHT OFF WITHOUT WILLPOWER WITH FOODS THAT NATURALLY CURB YOUR APPETITE AND *BURN UP AN EXTRA 200 CALORIES A DAY!*

<u>THE G-INDEX DIET</u>

"ONE OF THE MOST SOUGHT-AFTER NEW WEIGHT-LOSS/HEALTH BOOKS."
           —*Newark Star-Ledger*

"RECOGNIZES THAT DIETERS HAVE DIFFERENT CONCERNS and that one 21-day plan won't help you eat properly over a lifetime . . . convincing physiological explanations for weight problems."
           —*New Woman*

"THE BASIC DIET ADVICE IS SOUND."
           —*USA Today*

"PEOPLE OUGHT TO BE ABLE TO LOSE WEIGHT COMFORTABLY and keep the pounds off permanently . . . some of the high G-index foods will really surprise you."
           —*Jewish Herald-Voice*

Please turn the page for more praise for
THE G-INDEX DIET . . .

ALSO BY RICHARD N. PODELL, M.D., F.A.C.P.

Doctor, Why Am I So Tired?
Primary Prevention of Coronary Heart Disease
Physician's Guide To Diabetic Patient Self-Management
Physician's Guide To Compliance In Hypertension

THE
G-INDEX
DIET

Control Your
Glucose Level
and Lose
Weight Now

RICHARD N. PODELL, M.D., F.A.C.P.,
and William Proctor

WARNER BOOKS

NEW YORK   BOSTON

This book contains numerous case histories. In order to preserve the privacy of the people involved, we have disguised their appearances, names, and personal stories, so that they are not identifiable. As with any diet book you should consult your health professional before commencing a nutritional regimen.

All information contained in this book regarding brand name products is based on research by the authors which is accurate as of June 30, 1992.

If you purchase this book without a cover you should be aware that this book may have been stolen property and reported as "unsold and destroyed" to the publisher. In such case neither the author nor the publisher has received any payment for this "stripped book."

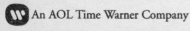

*This book is dedicated to the patients and staff
of the Overlook Center for Weight Management,
whose life experience and perseverance have helped
to make the G-Index Diet a reality.*

ACKNOWLEDGMENTS

Our most heartfelt thanks go to our literary agents Herb and Nancy Katz, whose professional wisdom and hard work were and remain indispensable. A special thanks is due to Nancy for her dedicated attention to culinary details.

Our editor, Susan Suffes, and her associates at Warner Books were unfailingly astute and supportive during the editorial process.

Several distinguished medical scientists have enhanced our understanding of the principles of weight control and metabolism through their publications, correspondence, or conversation. Our thanks to James Anderson, M.D.; George Blackburn, M.D.; George Bray, M.D.; Janette C. Brand, Ph.D.; Jeffrey Fisher, M.D.; David J. A. Jenkins, M.D., Ph.D.; Jean Mayer, Ph.D.; Judith Rodin, Ph.D.; Lawrence Stifler, Ph.D.; Albert Stunkard, M.D.; Thomas M.S. Wolever, Ph.D.

We thank Liz Fisher for her creative advice and enthusiasm. We appreciate the well-stocked shelves of King's Supermarket in Short Hills, New Jersey, and of Nature Food Centres in Livingston, New Jersey.

My thanks to Larry Hite for helping to sharpen my focus.

The staff and associates of Overlook Hospital and the Overlook Center for Weight Management have been extremely helpful. They include Jack Scharf; Lynn Lind, R.N.; Joyce Jukofsky, R.N.; Dolores Phillips; Shelly Beck; Beverly Licata, R.N.; Diane Powers; Mary Sealer; Nicholas Yatrakis, M.D.; Glen Landesman, M.D.; Ken Storch, M.D., Ph.D.; Ray Buch, M.D.; Janice Baker, M.D.; Gary Weine, M.D.; Ron Cobo; Connie F. Williams.

Our associates in private practice have provided unfailing support and loyalty: Jodi Geller, R.N.; Nancy Carter, R.N.; Linda DeCorso; Sandra Kearney; Andrea Shenocca; Peggy Stiner; Lori B. Katz, R.D.; Nora Cielo, M.S.; Jackie Massa; Mary Lou DiBari; Karen Croswell; Terry McGuirk; Robin Ford; Sally Karas, R.N.; Marjorie Knickerbocker, R.N.

A special thanks goes to my partner David K. Brown, M.D., for his enthusiasm and encouragement.

And of course, we are grateful to our families, who have supported us through this project: Patricia, Carrie, Lisa, and Tracy Podell; Pam and Michael Proctor; and Sergio, Matt, and Paul Burani.

CONTENTS

PART I

The Diet for Permanent Weight Loss

CHAPTER ONE

The Solution to the Seesaw Syndrome

Although there have been many breakthroughs recently in our understanding of diet and nutrition, a major element has been missing in most weight-loss programs: a way to take weight off and keep it off—*permanently*.

The dismal fact is that about 95 percent of people who lose weight gain most or all of it back in less than a year. In fact, millions of people on popular diet programs end up heavier than they were when they started. Perhaps *you* are one of these people, just as I was.

The recent emphasis on low-fat eating is certainly a step in the right direction. But a low-fat diet isn't the sole solution to the problem of weight gain after weight loss.

The main difficulty is that countless people *still remain hungry or dissatisfied* as they diet on a low-fat regimen, and also after they lose their excess weight. So, they slip off the diet, and before long, they put that weight right back on.

Up until a few years ago, I was subject to the "seesaw syndrome" or "yo-yo effect"—lay terms for the never-ending cycle of losing weight and then regaining it. Indeed, I lost thirty pounds on one low-fat diet, only to see my success disappear within months. Staying with the diet over the long term just took too much effort and willpower.

I almost never felt satisfied on a weight-loss program. Within hours of eating, my appetite would return with a vengeance. If a meal was delayed, I'd become lightheaded and jittery. I craved breads and crackers, and would gulp them down by the box when my resolve failed. As I began to eat more fat, I started to feel better. But I also regained my lost weight.

I sensed there had to be a better way, and I committed myself to finding it. Recalling lessons I had learned at the Harvard Medical School and the Harvard School of Public Health, I began an intensive, even obsessive exploration of the research that had been done on how specific foods alter our appetite control and influence how we feel.

Soon, I found the answer—the missing piece in the dieting puzzle. Specifically, I put together a food program based on the concept of the Glycemic Index (a rating system indicating how different foods affect the rise in blood sugar).

As powerful as the concept is, the basic premise is simple: Foods that have a *low* Glycemic Index (GI) are best for dieters because they promote a slow, moderate rise in blood sugar and insulin after a meal—factors which help keep hunger in check. These same factors also encourage the body to dissolve body fat by converting it into energy.

In contrast, *high* GI foods cause sudden, unstable swings in blood sugar, first with very high sugar and insulin surges, then with a crash of the sugar toward excessively low levels. The end result is increased appetite and irritability—and a greater tendency to convert food calories into body fat.

In short, the goal of the dieter is to build a food plan around *low* Glycemic Index foods. This way, hunger is minimized, and there is less tendency to overeat. Consequently, the dieter can continue to lose weight—or to maintain an ideal weight once the excess pounds have been lost.

This G-Index Diet, as I call it, has worked beautifully for me. I lost my excess 25 pounds in less than three months, and I didn't gain it back. As the medical director of the Overlook Center for Weight Management in Springfield, New Jersey (a program of Overlook Hospital, a teaching affiliate of the Columbia University College of Physicians and Surgeons), I also have put hundreds of my patients on the diet. It's worked as well for most of them as it has for me. They've taken the pounds off. Just as important, they haven't put them back on. Now, people who have been struggling with weight fluctuations can achieve stable weight reduction *permanently* through the G-Index program.

Here are a number of other exciting, compelling features of this revolutionary diet:

- The 21-day menus—including detailed recipes, shopping lists, and step-by-step instructions—are set up to make your dieting job as easy as possible. There's nothing to figure out. Almost everything has been done for you— except the eating!
- The program uses food—not a special liquid solution or other short-term dietary elixir—to help you eliminate excess weight.
- You can actually *increase* your caloric intake—and at the same time lose more weight than through deprivation.
- The diet is based on a well-researched, thoroughly documented, but often overlooked scientific fact: *Not all carbohydrates are equal for purposes of losing weight.*

Some carbohydrates, which I call the "bad" diet foods, actually increase your hunger. Carrots in quantity will increase your hunger. So will popcorn, along with honey, baked potatoes, oat bran flakes, most whole wheat breads, shredded wheat, watermelon, raisins, and lima beans.

In contrast, the "good" diet foods, which we describe in detail later in this book, are not that way simply because of their low caloric value, though obviously my diet is a controlled-calorie one. Rather, they are good because the body uses them to actually regulate hunger through a metabolic process that has been known in medical circles for decades. The concept just hasn't been applied to ordinary weight-loss diets until now.

The G-Index approach is entirely consistent with the low-fat, low-cholesterol, high-fiber principles demanded by recent medical and nutritional research. But this diet features a *strategic use of fats*. Specifically, certain fats, such as cheeses or peanut butter, eaten at the right time and in limited amounts with the right combination of other foods, not only help you feel more satisfied—they also promote better weight control.

Selecting the best foods for weight loss and designing a daily G-Index Diet are simple matters for people who use the food ratings, food exchanges, and model menus and recipes contained in this book.

In the following pages, you'll learn how to move beyond the commonplace and often erroneous wisdom of weight loss. You'll be shown not only how to lose those extra pounds, but also how to cure the hunger problem and end the seesaw syndrome forever.

HOW DOES THE G-INDEX DIET WORK?

After you eat, the level of sugar (glucose) rises in your bloodstream. Some foods—those with a high Glycemic Index—make the blood sugar increase more quickly and to a higher level than other foods. This rise in blood sugar leads to a corresponding sharp rise in insulin, which the body releases to regulate the blood sugar.

Unfortunately, that flood of insulin has negative side effects. High insulin levels stimulate the appetite by directly triggering the brain's appetite center. Furthermore, excess insulin can cause the blood sugar to "crash," setting off a chain of hormonal events that lead to irritability, fatigue, and even more hunger.

So a process that begins with a *rise* ends with a *fall*—and with a heightened craving for food. As a result, your hunger intensifies and your body begins to insist, "I need more to eat—*now!*" Overwhelming hunger takes over, and overeating results.

There's also another weight-control connection: *Insulin influences the ability of the body to burn calories*. When insulin levels are high, fewer calories are burned and more calories are transformed into fat. Conversely, when insulin levels are low, *more* calories are burned, fewer calories turn into fat—and body weight tends to decrease.

To make the best use of this phenomenon, a wise dieter must learn to identify and choose foods with a low Glycemic Index (GI). That's the secret to keeping blood sugar stable, insulin low, and hunger in check. In this book, comprehensive food listings and GI values for different foods have been included to assist you in selecting the best hunger-averting foods.

Among other things, you will learn how to apply principles like these:

* *Not all sugars are alike*. Fructose (the sugar in fruits) and lactose (milk sugar) are excellent low G-Index foods. Even table sugar (sucrose) is not as bad as has often been supposed. For example, it doesn't drive up the Glycemic Index as quickly as do some other sugars, most breads, or many breakfast cereals.

  On the other hand, honey is terrible. With its high Glycemic Index, honey drives up blood sugar and, as a consequence, draws insulin to a high level. This action paves the way for a crash in blood sugar and intense hunger pangs.

* *Some fat can help promote weight loss*. Every responsible, knowledgeable physician these days advocates a low-fat diet to keep blood cholesterol down, cancer risk at a minimum, and excess weight off.

  But there's an important variation on the low-fat thesis. Using *small* amounts of fats *prescriptively*, at well-chosen times during the day, actually can help stave off hunger. The reason? A limited amount of fat taken at the right time during a meal or as a snack can prevent the body from craving high-calorie between-meal or bedtime snacks.

* *Low GI foods provide the dieter with a ''200-calorie advantage'' in losing weight*. In effect, low GI foods raise the body's metabolism by about 8 percent because they are able to keep insulin levels low. I call this edge the ''200-calorie advantage'' because that's the average number of extra calories that can be burned each day *if* you choose more foods with a low GI.

This means that an overweight patient on the G-Index Diet can lose 15 pounds or more, even if he or she continues to consume the same number of calories! That's because the diet raises the body's metabolic rate and stimulates a more rapid burning of calories.

WHO SHOULD USE THE G-INDEX DIET?

As I've already indicated, the G-Index Diet has two major uses. First, you can *lose excess weight* simply by eating more foods with a lower Glycemic Index, even without lowering your daily intake of calories! Second, you can use the GI approach to *maintain lower weight* achieved initially through liquid diets or other weight-reduction programs.

I've discovered in my clinical practice that people with nearly every type of dieting problem can be helped by the G-Index program. These include:

- *People who hate to go on diets because they become almost intolerably ill-tempered or anxious.* The G-Index Diet has proved to be an ideal program to *lower* anxiety and irritability. When blood sugar crashes after the intake of high GI foods, the body releases adrenaline to limit the drop in sugar. The extra adrenaline is one of the factors that make hungry people edgy, jumpy, and angry. By keeping blood sugar more stable, an individual can ward off many attacks of anxiety and irritability.

- *Dieters who are making the transition to regular food from a low-calorie liquid diet.* For many of these patients, the return to solid food heralds the beginning of unstoppable weight gain. Yet I have successfully used liquid diets, followed by a permanent G-Index Diet, with patients needing to lose 50 pounds or more. They have continued to maintain their lower weight because the "natural" G-Index Diet has regulated their blood sugar, short-circuited their hunger surges, and allowed a choice of satisfying foods.

- *People who have managed to reduce down to within 10 to 20 pounds of their desired weight, but who somehow can't make it the rest of the way.* This situation, which confronted a woman named Sally, is typical of hundreds of people who have succeeded on our weight-loss program.

Sally—Whose Last 15 Pounds Were the Hardest

Sally had been on a diet for as long as she could remember. At 5-feet, 3-inches, her desired weight was 120 pounds, but she consistently tipped the scales at between 135 and 140. She constantly counted calories and tried one weight-loss program after another. But nothing worked. Granted, she would sometimes manage to lose about 5 pounds, but then she would gain it right back.

A person with tremendous self-discipline, Sally was very careful about what she ate. Often, she'd have just coffee and a few crackers for breakfast. But then, she would snack later in the morning on whole wheat bread, carrots, and low-fat meats like turkey and lean beef. Sometimes, she would even try a baked potato or some watermelon.

Obviously, she wasn't eating junk foods. In fact, many of the items on her diet were consistent with most diet programs because her meals were low in calories and fats. But that wasn't enough to keep the weight off because Sally constantly had to fight feelings of hunger, and like most of us, she eventually lost the battle.

Her problem was that she was following religiously the traditional weight-loss wisdom that says all that's necessary is to keep calories and fats to a minimum. Yet that *isn't* enough for a *permanent* program. Those old, established dietary ideas didn't prevent her from becoming ravenous within hours of a meal or snack. As a consequence, she ate so many "diet foods" that her weight regularly stayed 15 to 20 pounds above her target.

After taking a careful medical history, I performed a complete physical and found that Sally's metabolism was a little on the low side. This made it especially difficult for her to lose those last 15 pounds. But the real problem was her diet. An analysis revealed that Sally's carbohydrates were not well chosen. She ate only modest amounts of low Glycemic Index foods and kept herself going with the *wrong*, high GI foods. Breads, carrots, and watermelon were her undoing! All of these foods trigger high blood sugar and insulin. Ironically, even her pure protein snacks—turkey and lean beef—were bad choices because pure protein eaten without other foods stimulates insulin as much as pure sugar. As a result, her hunger stayed high and she failed to lose weight.

So I put her on the G-Index Diet, with these specific recommendations: A snack of sliced pears and apples (or strawberries in season) late in the morning or in the middle of the afternoon would abolish her hunger pangs far better than either crackers, bread, or turkey, and help her feel far less famished by mealtime. Also, a couple of thin slices of skim-milk goat cheese would help if she felt the need for anything a couple of hours after her evening meal. Lastly, throughout her daily menus, she would exchange high GI foods for low GI fare.

Free from the vicious GI cycle, Sally lost 8 pounds in six months without really dieting. Though she eats as much as before, her food selections have improved her metabolism by allowing her body to burn more calories. She's never hungry, yet the pounds continue to come off. From the look of things, Sally will continue to lose weight until she reaches her goal.

HOW CAN THE G-INDEX DIET WORK FOR YOU?

In the following sections of this book, I will lead you systematically through the information you'll need to apply the Glycemic Index concept to your own diet program. Here are some of the highlights.

The Scientific Basis

Medical investigators, especially those concerned with diabetes, have uncovered information with important implications for *all* dieters. Among other things, you'll see how:

- Foods that stimulate insulin surges in the body can cause people to eat 60 to 70 percent more calories at the following meal.
- People who consume foods relatively high in glucose (such as white bread, most commercial whole wheat bread, and raisins) eat an average of 200 calories more at the next meal than those who eat fructose (a sugar found in most fruits).
- All high-fiber foods are not equal as far as dieters are concerned. For example, pineapple, instant or one-minute oatmeal, oat bran flakes, and most whole wheat breads—even those containing relatively high amounts of fiber—may nevertheless stimulate hunger. In contrast, hunger can be suppressed with apples, orange juice, non-sugared yogurt, regular oatmeal, whole-grain rye crackers, 100 percent stone-ground whole wheat bread, and European-style pumpernickel bread.
- Some low-fiber foods—such as pasta (even pasta based on white flour)—may actually be better for dieters than certain high-fiber foods, such as most commercial whole wheat breads and breakfast cereals.
- Certain ethnic cuisines, like Indian and Greek, which often contain lentils and other low GI foods, have proved to help dieters avoid hunger pangs.
- Low GI foods (good for dieting) can be mixed with modest quantities of high GI foods (worse for dieting, though they may satisfy certain tastes) without losing their hunger-reducing effect.
- Combining *small* amounts of fat with high GI foods will reduce the appetite-stimulating effect of high GI foods.
- Eating a low GI snack two hours before dinner can reduce your appetite at supper. Also, eating low GI foods at dinner can reduce your appetite at breakfast the next morning.
- The best sweetener for hot or cold drinks is fructose, a fruit sugar that is available in most supermarkets. It's also acceptable to use *small* amounts of sucrose, or table sugar say, one or two teaspoons. That's because sucrose has a moderate Glycemic Index. Please don't overdo it.

but modest quantities of sugar are actually less damaging to your diet than are higher GI carbohydrates such as most commercial bread.

- There is evidence that low GI foods, such as spaghetti and dried beans, reduce the level of blood cholesterol and triglycerides.
- Eating three large meals a day stimulates insulin production—and hunger—more than small, more frequent feedings.
- Substituting low for high G-Index foods can increase your metabolism and improve your body's ability to remove fat and burn calories.

After you've been introduced to such scientific findings and concepts, you'll next see how they have been applied successfully to help a wide variety of dieters.

A Diet for All Seasons—And All Sorts of Weight Problems

We explore how people with various needs have succeeded in losing weight and keeping it off by employing the scientific principles on which the G-Index Diet is based. The case studies include the following types of dieters:

- People who have lost 50 pounds or more on liquid protein diets—and then have used the G-Index Diet to achieve successful long-term weight maintenance.
- People who have lost modest amounts of weight—averaging about 20 pounds—using only the G-Index Diet.
- People who have been totally frustrated by not being able to take off—and keep off—an extra 5 to 7 pounds around the middle and hips. They broke through this weight barrier by employing the Glycemic Index approach.
- People who have been fighting excess pounds since childhood.
- Sweets and salt cravers who have been unable to conquer their drives and stay on a long-term weight-loss regimen.

- People who have suffered chronically from the seesaw syndrome—with many ups and downs on different programs—until they went on the G-Index Diet.
- People who have used the G-Index Diet to conquer emotional problems that often emerge during a weight-reduction program, such as increased irritability and anxiety.

As you learn how these people have accomplished long-term weight loss, you'll be introduced to some practical techniques and tactics that will help you succeed on your own weight-reduction program.

Tactics to Protect Yourself from Hunger

A number of practical approaches to weight loss and maintenance have worked for my patients—and should also work for you—in the battle against the seesaw syndrome. For example, you'll be introduced to such techniques as:

- Eating low GI foods at your most vulnerable and tempting times of the day, such as late morning, late afternoon, and late evening.
- Using small portions of fat to promote weight loss (though the total fat consumed each day will usually stay below 25 percent of total calories).
- Identifying and always keeping on hand four or five favorite low GI foods to stave off hunger.
- Intelligent eating plans for restaurant dining.
- Ways to translate many of the GI scientific concepts into practical meal planning in the kitchen.

G-Index Diet Menus, Recipes, and Food Exchange Lists

The detailed meals and recipes presented in Chapter Five are the heart of the program. You'll be presented with a model food plan designed as follows:

1. Recommended foods have been selected according to their low rating on the Glycemic Index. These low GI foods provide a slow, steady input of sugar into the blood and avoid disruptive swings in blood sugar and insulin, which can trigger hunger.

2. For ease of evaluation and selection, both recommended and nonrecommended foods have been classified in groups numbering 1 through 4. Foods that are in categories 1 and 2 are low on the Glycemic Index and should be preferred by all dieters. Those in categories 3 or 4 should generally be avoided, though I've allowed for some strategic "cheating" on occasion.

3. Fat intake is low, usually constituting less than 25 percent of total calories each day. This guideline is consistent with current advice about keeping blood lipids, such as cholesterol, at a low level. Also, there is a need on any weight-loss diet to limit fats, which have more than twice as many calories as the same weight of either protein or carbohydrates.

4. The model menus involve three weeks of meals at different calorie levels, depending on whether you want to lose weight or maintain your present weight. People on the 1,200-calorie weight-loss plan can expect to lose 2 to 5 pounds per week, and do it on their own, without medical supervision. (Of course, people with liver or gall bladder problems, kidney disease, metabolic disorders, or other medical conditions should check with their doctor before making any changes in their nutritional programs.)

After the excess weight has been taken off, the 1,500 and 1,800-calorie menus will enable you to maintain the new, lower weight level that you've achieved. Guidelines help you choose the menus appropriate for your particular weight-control needs. To accommodate the demands of busy and varied schedules, there's also a program for restaurant eating.

5. The comprehensive food exchange lists in Chapter Eight have been set up so that you can adjust the model diets to your special tastes. Or using the low GI approach, you can employ the lists to design a completely different set of menus for yourself.

As with any weight-loss program, you should consult with your physician before embarking on the G-Index Diet.

Now, with this in mind, you're ready to take your first step: a look at how different individuals with different weight-loss problems and objectives have all succeeded on the G-Index Diet. If your experience is similar, you'll find that these real-life stories will soon lead you to a major, highly satisfying transformation in your life and your appearance.

CHAPTER TWO

A Diet for All Seasons

The G-Index Diet has been designed to work for *everyone* who needs to take pounds off—and keep them off. If you need to lose 5, 50, or 150 pounds, the program will meet your needs. Furthermore, the diet can help you overcome such diet-breakers as special food cravings, stress reactions, and the low self-esteem that often accompanies a loss of control over food.

To help you understand how the G-Index regimen works in different situations, consider the following weight-loss challenges.

CHALLENGE 1: A DIET FOR LIQUID PROTEIN USERS

Many dieters, especially those with 40 or more pounds to lose, rely on a liquid protein solution for fast initial weight loss. Unfortunately, these very same people frequently become victims of the seesaw syndrome, because when they go back on regular food, they lack an effective weight-maintenance plan. They begin to eat as they did before their diet, and their weight comes right back up, often to a heavier level than before they began the diet.

But this unfortunate mechanism that causes weight gain after weight loss isn't necessary. People who combine a liquid protein diet (which should always be pursued under medical supervision) with the G-Index Diet can take off a great deal of weight *and* keep it off. The experience of Lois, a former victim of yo-yo dieting, shows clearly how this combination solution can work.

Lois and the Liquid Solution

Lois, whose weight had risen to 240 pounds, had tried many diets and, on occasion, lost a great deal of weight. But she couldn't prevent the pounds from coming back. At 5-feet, 5-inches, her ideal body weight was in the 113- to 126-pound range, but her initial personal weight-loss goal was more modest. She said she would be quite content if she could just make it to 150 pounds "and stay there!"

The first decision I faced was what type of diet to use to help her get rid of those first 90 pounds. Speed is often essential in achieving a large weight loss because diets that take too long may lead to discouragement. So we selected a 600-calorie per day liquid protein diet that was designed to provide a weight loss of about 3 pounds a week, or 14 pounds per month.

Medical supervision is required for people consuming so few calories each day because of the risk of dehydration, mineral loss, gallstones, and other complications. But for those who stick with the program, the results are often fast and dramatic.

Lois was quite successful and managed to lose steadily an average of 4 pounds a week. One reason she lost more weight than many people on a liquid protein regimen is that she included regular walking in her program. Within six months, she had lost her 90 pounds, but it was at this point that her problems began.

Like many people who succeed on a liquid protein diet, she was thrilled with the weight loss but terrified when she considered returning to regular eating. She knew that she had never managed to keep weight off after a diet, and she feared the same failure would occur again.

The first week of regular eating was really a shocker. She gained 4 pounds while eating only 900 calories a day. The next week, she gained another 4 pounds despite eating only 1,200 calories a day. I explained that this was water weight; it was really nothing to worry about.

But during the next eight weeks, she continued to gain about 1 pound a week on what was supposed to be a 1,500-calorie per day diet. Why? She kept getting hungry and couldn't stop eating. She experienced cravings for bread, potatoes, and almost any kind of between-meal snack.

Our dietitian checked Lois's food program and found that she fit neatly into the high Glycemic Index pattern: She was overdosing on breads, caffeine, raisins, popcorn, and baked potatoes. I encouraged her to emphasize low Glycemic Index foods such as fruits, vegetables, certain breads like pumpernickel, 100 percent whole-grain rye crackers, and dairy products like skim milk and nonsugared yogurt.

The first week of adjusting to this low Glycemic Index diet provoked some anxiety in Lois. She worried that the approach would fail, as had all the others. But gradually her confidence increased as she noticed she was less hungry. Also, she found she was no longer "dieting." In other words, she didn't have to turn her back on tasty foods while fighting off hunger. Instead, she ate even more of the low GI items she liked, and as a result, she seemed constantly to feel satisfied or "full."

To be sure, holiday parties were a strain at first, and she occasionally slipped back into her old high Glycemic Index habits. But after about three months on the low GI program, she found that even when she occasionally overindulged, she could easily get right back on her regular eating plan.

Lois, like most of my other patients, discovered that after the first month or so, deviations from a low GI eating program are usually self-correcting. At first, people reexperience their hypoglycemic symptoms of hunger and irritability. But, with the information they've acquired about the Glycemic Index of various foods, they recognize what's happening to them. In most cases, they immediately seek out the proper, low GI foods to remedy the problem.

It's now eighteen months since Lois finished her liquid protein fast and embarked on the G-Index Diet. She has actually lost *extra* weight and has dipped below 150. In other words, the G-Index approach is not only helping her maintain a lower weight but is actually bringing about further weight loss.

Lois's success is unusual for people not on the G-Index Diet, in that we generally regard a weight-control effort to be successful if the person can keep off 80 percent of the lost weight over about a two-year period. She has gone well beyond that goal. Also, she has strengthened her program by walking three miles a day, five days a week, and by attending group reinforcement sessions once a month.

As for her diet, Lois consumes an average of 2,000 calories per day—only 600 less than when she weighed 240 pounds! But now she makes very different food choices by concentrating heavily on foods with a low Glycemic Index.

Lois's experience can easily serve as a diet pattern for many others who have taken off prodigious amounts of weight on a liquid protein diet and then wonder what will come next. What comes next *must* be the G-Index Diet, or the seesaw syndrome is sure to kick in and destroy all those hard-earned weight-loss achievements.

CHALLENGE 2:
A DIET FOR CRAVERS

One of the most vicious diet-breakers is a craving that develops for a particular type of food. All resolutions and good intentions go out the window when the drive strikes for something salty or sweet, or perhaps for food of a certain texture, such as crunchy crackers.

The G-Index Diet isn't a panacea for all cravings. But using the principles of food selection described in this book, you can launch an effective counterattack against the temptations associated with eating a wide variety of foods.

Sam and Carbohydrate Cravings

Perhaps the easiest temptation to handle with the G-Index Diet is a *general* craving for carbohydrates. When some people get hungry, they satisfy that hunger by consuming practically any carbohydrate, such as bread, raisins, pasta, or fruit. The food doesn't have to be sweet or salty, nor does it have to be anything specific. All that's required is *any* carbohydrate.

Sam was in this category. A fifty-five-year-old executive, he was a regular jogger in good health, with a relatively low cholesterol level and normal blood pressure. But Sam was dissatisfied with his appearance because he was consistently 8 to 15 pounds above his ideal weight of 155 pounds. He just couldn't seem to get down to his target and stay there. On a number of occasions, Sam had made it down to 157 or 158, but then he would go right back up to between 163 and 170.

A rather disciplined person, Sam could stick to a calorie-counting regimen for three to four weeks to lose the extra weight. His usual strategy was to eliminate completely breads, desserts, and between-meal snacks. He had determined that by cutting out these foods, he would lower his caloric intake enough to lose about 2 to 3 pounds a week.

Although Sam often became hungry before a meal, he was able to hold out until it was time to eat. Then when he sat down to his meal, he would *continue* his disciplined ways by refusing "forbidden" foods such as breads.

Unfortunately, he could maintain this willpower only for about three weeks. One of Sam's latest dieting forays is typical. After he had lost about 8 pounds, he began to congratulate himself on his success. He decided it was time to reward himself with some of the foods he had eliminated from his diet. So he ate some raisins and crackers for a snack in the middle of the afternoon. Then when he sat down at his very next meal, he consumed an entire loaf of French bread. Sam's diet effectively was demolished at this point! He engaged in a series of carbohydrate binges, and his weight shot back up to 170 pounds.

Sam's problem was that in the years since childhood, he had developed a general craving for carbohydrates. The foods didn't have to be sweet, nor did they need to be salty. The key requirement was that the nearest carbohydrate within reach go into his mouth.

This meant that at a regular meal, he first attacked the bread, which was most likely to be the only food on the table when he took his seat. For snacks, he would typically buy a carbonated, sweetened drink with a small box of raisins, a packaged piece of cake, or perhaps a candy bar. Then when dinner time arrived, he would eat even more of his normal meal than he usually did. The pounds built up until he launched his next period of disciplined dieting.

The G-Index solution to Sam's problem was relatively simple. All he had to do was become better informed about the nature of the carbohydrates he was consuming at the beginning of his binge. Then he would be in a position to make wiser choices.

During a series of diet counseling sessions, Sam learned the facts about the foods he was binging on when he went off his diet—the bread, cake, raisins, and glucose-laden soft drinks and candy bars. They weren't satisfying his hunger; they were actually *triggering* his appetite.

With the exception of desserts, these foods weren't so high in calories, but they *were* high on the Glycemic Index. In other words, they were threatening his appetite and his diet. Three important things were happening in his body when he ate high GI foods: (1) his blood sugar rose rapidly; (2) large amounts of insulin were released by his pancreas to counter the high sugar level; and (3) his blood sugar crashed to a low level, triggering a discharge of adrenaline, a potent stress-inducing adrenal gland hormone. A side effect of this roller-coaster effect was stimulation of his appetite beyond normal bounds.

Sam, then, was simply choosing the *wrong* carbohydrates

to satisfy his appetite. He got off on the wrong foot with his afternoon snacks, which were high on the Glycemic Index, and these began to stimulate his hunger. Then he made matters worse by wolfing down all that bread at his evening meal. As a result, Sam ate extra helpings and wasn't satisfied until he had polished off a dessert.

The solution for this carbohydrate craver was *not* to give up carbohydrates but, rather, to pick carbos with a low rating on the Glycemic Index. Sam was advised to choose his afternoon snacks more wisely, since that's where his massive hunger urges began. He began to eat a nonsugared low-fat or nonfat yogurt snack and a piece of fresh fruit in the middle of the day. Any dairy food and most fruits are low on the Glycemic Index because these foods are converted relatively slowly into sugar in the blood. As a result, Sam's new snacks caused no blood sugar surge, no precipitous rise in insulin level, no plunge in blood sugar, *and* no unusual increase in appetite.

By the time Sam was ready for his evening meal, he was less hungry than he had been eating a snack of raisins, cake, candy, or soft drink. Still, he didn't take any chances trying to stare down a loaf of bread on the table. Instead, when he arrived home he immediately ate a salad or half a grapefruit, or ordered a similar dish if he was at a restaurant. Vegetables and fresh fruit—especially fruit like grapefruit—are low on the Glycemic Index. Consequently, they don't act as an appetite trigger.

Now Sam was equipped to lose that extra weight and keep it off. He went on one of his commendable, well-disciplined programs again, but this time the challenge was much less. He didn't have to eliminate his snacks; he just chose different ones, including more fresh fruit and yogurt. Also, at his regular meal he concentrated on foods that are low on the Glycemic Index. His favorites included pasta shells, pita bread, sweet potatoes, kidney beans, and extra helpings of vegetables. By balancing his diet with carbohydrates that are low, rather than high, on the Glycemic Index, Sam took the edge off his appetite—and was able to keep off the pounds that he lost.

Beth and a Craving for Crunchiness

I've encountered people who really don't care that much what they nibble on, so long as it's crunchy. Beth, a thirty-five-year-old mother, was a "crunchy craver" who weighed 182 pounds when she came to our weight-loss center for help. She really needed to lose weight—not just for the sake of appearance but also because both her cholesterol and blood pressure were elevated.

Specifically, Beth's blood pressure was 140/90 millimeters of mercury (mmHg), or borderline hypertensive (normal is below 140/90). Her total cholesterol was about 320 milligrams per deciliter (mg/dl), a level far too high for good health. (The American Heart Association recommends that total cholesterol be below 200.) Put another way, Beth's borderline blood pressure and high cholesterol level put her at high risk for heart disease and stroke. Yet most people like Beth can lower their blood pressure and cholesterol level—*and* their risk of suffering these diseases—by losing weight. That was the goal Beth set for herself during our counseling sessions.

Beth did a commendable job by losing 45 pounds in less than four months on a medically supervised 800-calorie per day diet. Her regimen consisted of a commercial liquid food supplement for breakfast, lunch, and snacks, and a simple, planned 400-calorie evening meal. But after losing 45 pounds, her weight started to creep back up. By the end of a year, she had regained 15 pounds and seemed well on her way back to her old level of obesity.

Fortunately, Beth came in for intensive counseling, during which we identified the culprit: her craving for crunchiness. In the course of an extensive interview, she revealed that the main thing that caused her to go off any diet was the temptation of foods that crunch, especially starchy snacks such as breadsticks, crackers, cookies, and bread crusts. It was apparent that Beth wasn't primarily drawn to sweet foods, nor was she crazy about salty things, nor was she addicted to soft breads or other spongy items like pancakes. She just had to feel the crunch in her mouth!

Yet Beth's craving for crunchiness didn't extend to vegetables or fruits. The food had to be a breadlike starch, or the appeal just wasn't present. Unfortunately, all the foods that Beth said she desired were high on the Glycemic Index. This explained her tendency to gain back those lost pounds; as she nibbled on the crunchy, high GI things, they triggered her appetite and she ate too much.

The challenge was to find foods that had a low GI and yet would satisfy Beth's need for a crunchy, breadlike texture. It took a lot of thought and discussion. She rejected every fruit and vegetable I suggested, and also said that a dairy product such as yogurt wouldn't do. The fruits and vegetables didn't melt in her mouth with that ''yeasty'' aftertaste, and obviously the yogurt didn't crunch at all.

Finally, we found some possibilities in toast. Pumpernickel bread and coarse whole-grain rye bread are relatively low on the Glycemic Index. When toasted, they satisfied much of Beth's need for a crunchy texture. But still, she said, she needed something more—a little more interesting taste, so we suggested that she use some low-calorie jelly. That was all she required: a half-piece of pumpernickel toast with jelly in the afternoon, followed by a plum or peach. The small amount of toast met her crunchy craving and allowed her to enjoy either fruit, both of which have a very low GI.

To broaden her range of snacks, Beth continued to search for crunchy foods that are low on the Glycemic Index. At this point, she has found candidates in the cracked and sprouted-wheat forms of whole wheat bread, which may be found in health food stores. She also selected toasted pockets of pita bread, and 100 percent whole-grain rye crackers, such as Ry Krisp and Wasa Bread.

Charlie and a Craving for Salt or Sugar

Charlie, a warehouse foreman in his mid-thirties, weighed nearly 280 pounds when he decided he had to lose weight. He went on a medically supervised liquid protein diet, and after many months his weight dropped to just under 190.

His goal was 180 pounds, which seemed about right for his medium-heavy frame and 6-foot, 1-inch height.

Because he had almost reached his objective, Charlie stopped using the liquid protein and began to eat regular food. But in just a few weeks his weight began to climb up again. When he passed the 220 mark, he came in for some counseling, and here's what emerged from our conversations.

Charlie reported that his self-esteem and his energy levels had *decreased* after he had gone off the liquid protein diet. That didn't make sense to me at first, because he had been taking in only 600 calories a day on the liquid protein program. His regular-food diet, in contrast, provided 1,200 calories, which should have given him *more* energy.

Further discussions revealed some of the reasons for Charlie's physical and emotional responses, however. For one thing, he noted that he had a craving for both sugar and salt, and he felt that the liquid protein program had *cleansed* his system by eliminating those factors. But there was some sugar and salt in the regular foods he began to eat after he completed the liquid protein fast. Consequently, he found himself drawn back into a salt-sugar cycle that increased his appetite and resulted in high calorie consumption and large weight gains.

"If I have something sweet, a lot of times I want something salty afterward," he explained. "Then, after that, I want something sweet again. So I might have a piece of cake, and that would make me want some potato chips. But the potato chips would cause me to eat more cake."

Charlie described a classic salt-sugar cycle that grips many people and destroys countless diets. He said that the problem wasn't just that his appetite increased; rather, he felt "crazed" and unable to stop once he began to alternate the sweet and salty foods. He actually began to consume so much that, by my estimates, he more than doubled his calorie intake, from the 1,200-calorie per day diet goal to actual consumption of 2,500 to 3,500 calories per day.

As we talked, though, Charlie noted that fruits, which also contain sugar, didn't set off the cycle. Neither did spaghetti. In other words, he confirmed what I already knew about the G-Index Diet. The salty and sweet foods he had been eating—

such as cake, potato chips, and pretzels—are *high* on the Glycemic Index. They stimulated his appetite and set off the seesaw syndrome which caused his weight to climb again.

In contrast, the fruits and spaghetti he sometimes ate are *low* on the Glycemic Index. They digest more slowly and cause only moderate increases in blood sugar over a longer period of time. These foods don't trigger a salt-sugar hunger cycle, and they also don't cause any sharp increase in fatigue or appetite.

The fatigue Charlie felt while on the higher-calorie diet was easily explained by looking at how his body used the high GI foods. Once consumed, they released a sharp surge of glucose into his bloodstream, accompanied by a surge of insulin. Then there would be a crash of the blood sugar to low levels, along with a release of extra adrenaline to keep the sugar from dropping too far. The process typically causes fatigue, irritability, and an overwhelming sense of hunger.

To understand more precisely how the different types of sugars operate in Charlie's body, as well as in your own body, let's consider briefly some key facts about sugar in our diet.

Why All Sugars Are Not Alike

A savvy dieter needs to be aware of the impact of four different kinds of sugar on the body, and how they affect a person's attempt to lose weight and keep it off. These sugars are glucose, fructose, lactose, and sucrose. Granted, there are many other types of sugar, but if you just understand these four, you'll have all the weapons you need to deal with the sugar in your life.

Glucose is the main type of sugar in your bloodstream. Also, glucose is added to many foods, such as desserts, to make them sweeter to the taste. Corn syrup, honey, maple sugar, and molasses contain large amounts of glucose. The carbohydrates you eat—such as breads, vegetables, and pastas—are changed by your digestive system into glucose for processing by your body. High GI foods are transformed into blood glucose quickly; low GI foods are altered more slowly.

The second main type of sugar, *fructose*, is found mainly in fruits, though it may also be added to foods as a sweetener. This sugar doesn't change easily into glucose because of the different way the body processes it. Therefore, eating fructose does not cause a major increase in blood sugar levels and does not provoke a large insulin response. That's why most fruit and fruit juices rate desirably low on the Glycemic Index scale. (One exception: Those diabetics who are in poor control of their blood sugar do have a large blood sugar rise after eating fructose, and so the G-Index Diet is not appropriate for them. Their priority is first to get their blood sugar working properly in treatments supervised by their physician.)

The third type of sugar, *lactose*, is found in milk products, including yogurt. Like fructose, it is metabolized slowly into the body through a process that is quite different from that involved with glucose.

Foods that contain a great deal of glucose, or which convert rapidly into glucose, tend to be high on the Glycemic Index. As a result, they aren't good diet foods. Those that have more fructose and lactose are low on the Glycemic Index. Experiments have shown that low GI foods enhance the burning of calories more than glucose. Also, these low GI foods cause only moderate elevation in levels of blood sugar or insulin. Consequently, foods with fructose and lactose tend to be superior diet foods.

The fourth type of sugar is *sucrose*, which is ordinary table sugar. A modest amount of sucrose is acceptable for those on a weight-reduction diet, since its chemical composition causes its Glycemic Index to be *higher* than that of fructose, lactose, or other low GI foods, but *lower* than that of white bread, honey, or pure glucose. So putting a *small* amount of sucrose (1 or 2 teaspoons = 15–30 calories) in a hot drink or other food won't harm your dieting efforts *so long as most of your foods are low on the Glycemic Index*.

Finally, here are a couple of other points about sugar that will prove helpful to your diet:

1. According to the *American Journal of Clinical Nutrition*, participants in a 1988 study tended to eat considerably

more food after taking in glucose than after taking in fructose. On average, the after-glucose people consumed 200 more calories than the after-fructose group. Hence, a low Glycemic Index diet, with an emphasis on fructose over glucose, could make a 200-calorie difference every day! That adds up to more than 15 pounds a year.

2. Even if you consume foods that contain a reasonable amount of fructose, you must examine your labels to be sure they are not outweighed by a similar or greater amount of glucose. For example, in one study, a non-dairy tofu-based frozen dessert was found to have 24 percent fructose, but it also had 29 percent glucose. That is enough glucose to give this food a high ranking on the Glycemic Index—and to ensure that people eating it experience a surge in blood sugar and insulin—and severe hunger pangs!

To sum up, then, your goal as a dieter should be to choose those foods that are low in glucose but higher in fructose or lactose. Clearly, not all sugars are alike—at least not for those who hope to lose weight!

The solution to Charlie's craving was rather simple. He focused on breaking the sugar-salt cycle in his eating, in part by selecting good sugars and avoiding bad ones. He learned about the G-Index and used the menus, recipes, and other information that would help him select and eat foods low on the Glycemic Index. Within a week, Charlie's weight increases stopped. Now on the way back to his original target, he tips the scales at just under 200 pounds.

Lydia: Is There an Answer for Chocolate Cravers?

Some food cravings are extremely difficult for certain dieters to handle, and one of the worst is the need for chocolate.

Lydia, a hospital administrator in her mid-forties, was a chocolate craver. She weighed 128 pounds but wanted to get down to an ideal weight of 112. At the higher weight she said she felt "dumpy" and "unattractive" and "tired all the time." Her goal was to lose 16 pounds—an amount that was small enough not to justify the use of a liquid protein supplement.

She went on a weight-loss program that is offered in various centers around the country, and she quickly began to shed the pounds. In addition to restricting her calories, she embarked on a walking-jogging aerobic exercise program, which aided in the weight loss. But when she got down to about 116, her weight started to climb again.

What was the problem? For one thing, she stopped doing her exercises regularly. But there was more to it than that. Whenever Lydia went on a diet, she would stop eating all chocolate. For a couple of days, she would actually experience withdrawal symptoms, probably from caffeine-like chemicals in the chocolate. But she would be able to get along just fine for a while without the chocolate, and the pounds would melt away. Then, when Lydia had nearly reached her weight goal, she would usually decide to reward herself by having just one piece of chocolate. "But I can't have just one piece," she confessed. "It just triggers something in me. I'll play a game with myself, saying, 'I'm just going to have one piece,' and that's all I'll take at first. But then I'll walk back to the kitchen and take another piece, and another."

The large majority of calories in chocolate candy come from fat, and fat contains about twice as many calories as an equal quantity of carbohydrate or protein. As a result, Lydia greatly increased her calorie intake and gained weight when she went on these chocolate binges.

Also, her hunger for other foods was stimulated by the chocolate. One reason was probably a caffeine-like substance called theobromine, which along with certain other chemicals in chocolate can overstimulate the appetite control center in the brain. Also, Lydia often chose chocolate-covered pastries, which were very high on the Glycemic Index. As you know, such foods trigger the glucose-insulin reactions in the blood and also increase the appetite.

In the end, Lydia found that she had to go cold turkey on the chocolate. In contrast, some people who are *not* chocolate cravers can eat a square or two of chocolate at the end of the meal, and this practice may actually *help* them lose weight, since the minimal quantity of fat in foods such as a small amount of cheese or chocolate can stave off hunger for a relatively long period. I advise some dieters to incorporate a small amount of chocolate at the end of a meal to help them maintain their program.

But Lydia wasn't in this category. As a chocolate craver, she had to cut it out completely to keep her weight off. She's currently finding significant success in adding small amounts of other fats, such as cheese, to her diet. The presence of some fat, though it doesn't tantalize her in the same way chocolate does, reduces the drive to eat chocolate. But in the last analysis, Lydia has to stay away from her most dangerous trigger food if she hopes to maintain her weight loss.

In most cases of food cravings, then, the G-Index Diet provides an excellent solution. In fact, for many cravers, it's the *only* solution that really works.

Now let's explore another serious dieting challenge: the tremendous obstacles that must be overcome by those who have been fighting obesity since childhood.

CHALLENGE 3: A DIET FOR LIFELONG OBESITY

A number of people I've worked with have been fighting obesity all their lives. They started getting fat when they were children, and the war against extra weight has been waged for decades, often with little success.

The G-Index Diet has proved an excellent response to the challenge of lifelong obesity.

Laura's Food Rewards

A working mother in her mid-thirties, Laura had been overweight since her days as a preschooler. "I was always motivated through food," she said. "My parents often said, 'If you'll be good, we'll give you a cookie.' " So an early childhood pattern conditioned her to believe that overeating, or eating sweet and fatty foods, was an appropriate reward for achievement, or a means to relieve personal frustration.

Eventually, her burgeoning weight problem thrust her into a vicious cycle. She didn't feel comfortable or adequate playing sports or exercising with the other children because she was overweight. Yet at the same time, she needed to engage in more vigorous activity to help burn up calories. As a result, she continued to put on weight until she topped 200 by the time she reached her twenties.

Those excess pounds, on a medium, 5-foot, 6-inch frame, caused her to feel constantly tired. She couldn't meet the needs of her demanding job and family life and still be in a good mood or have any energy left at the end of the day.

What Laura needed was a weight-loss program that would take off the pounds, and also a weight-maintenance strategy that would help her keep them off. She had not been able to lose more than about 20 pounds on any program before she would break her diet and regain the weight. One of her problems was that she disliked many of the liquid protein solutions, and found she couldn't stay on them long enough to lose the required weight. The temptations of her regular, high-calorie habits were too great.

When she began coming to our clinic, I placed Laura on a liquid protein diet, with the understanding that this was a short-term strategy. She would be able to switch to a regular-food diet after she had lost a designated number of pounds—a goal we set at 170, or about 30 pounds below her current weight. Then she would go on a G-Index Diet to lose another 30 pounds.

I knew that if she could get down to 140 pounds—a level she hadn't reached since she had been a child—she would have overcome a major obstacle. Furthermore, if she could *stay* on the G-Index Diet, and I was convinced that she could, she would have a good chance of at least maintaining her weight loss and even of losing extra pounds.

Laura succeeded in losing more than 30 pounds on the liquid protein regimen in only about two months, primarily because she knew she didn't have to lose *all* her excess poundage with this method. She had a manageable goal that she knew was within her reach, and she proceeded to meet it.

The second part of her strategy, the regular-food regimen, involved a little more thought and planning. She was now 168 pounds, and she could already begin to see the natural shape of her body emerging from the folds of fat. Her fear was that the seesaw syndrome would take over her life again, and she would quickly regain all her hard-lost weight.

But I assured her that this result wasn't necessary with the G-Index Diet. We embarked on several counseling sessions that first explored those low GI foods that she liked most. Remember, the G-Index Diet is a diet of wise selection, not a diet of denial. You don't have to give up all those great foods you love. It's just necessary to find favorite foods that reduce the surge of sugar and insulin in your blood and thus help you control your hunger.

We also investigated the foods that tended to trigger Laura's appetite—a process that led us to discuss a rather bizarre diet she had once tried. Laura recalled one diet in the past that involved eating large quantities of lettuce, carrots, pineapple, and watermelon. She lost some pounds on this diet, which she called the "watermelon-pineapple diet," but it left her with a periodic craving for bread. That's because pineapple, watermelon, and carrots in quantity are very high on the Glycemic Index, and tend to stimulate the appetite.

Laura broke this diet by consuming an entire loaf of white bread in one day. She fully intended to go back on the diet the next day, but the hunger triggered by the "diet" foods didn't allow that. Instead, she began to eat desserts and other forbidden dishes, and the pounds she had lost came right back.

I asked her if eating other fruit had the same impact on her appetite. She noted that oranges and pears were "definitely better" than pineapples and watermelon in holding down her hunger and allowing her to stay on her weight-loss program. In fact, one week while she was on her watermelon-pineapple diet, Laura had eaten daily helpings of oranges and pears whenever she needed a snack or dessert, and her craving for desserts or fatty dishes hadn't increased.

At first, when Laura switched to low G-Index choices, her diet progressed nicely and her appetite stayed in check. But as we slowly increased her caloric intake, she noticed significant weight gains.

"I was eating sensibly—lots of fruits and vegetables without overdoing it—but then I'd suddenly gain weight for no apparent reason," she said. "Sometimes, I'd add two or three pounds in a day, and that really scared me." The weight Laura gained as she modestly increased her food intake was mostly, if not all, fluid.

The Water Factor

All carbohydrates, including low G-Index choices, contain a great amount of water. More important, eating carbohydrates causes the body to hang on to water. (The same is true of eating salt.) The tendency for even a little extra carbohydrate to trigger water retention often produces large, though temporary, weight gains for up to three months.

No matter what is causing the additional pounds, gaining weight while you're eating sensibly can be a frustrating and terrifying experience for a dieter. But there is plenty of reason to stay calm, comfortable, and confident at this point. First, you'll gain back your water weight loss only once. Also, the tendency to hold on to water after weight loss is a temporary phenomenon. Your body's water-retention system gets back to normal in a short period.

A man named Bill, who was 380 pounds when he came to our center, is a good illustration of this water issue. He lost 140 pounds during seven months on a medically supervised, 800-calorie liquid diet. But during his first week off the liquid regimen, he began a low GI program consisting of 1,300 calories each day. That was well below the 2,800 break-even level we had established to enable him to maintain whatever weight he had lost. But still Bill gained 20 pounds. And the next week, he gained another 19 pounds.

He was beside himself. Sure that he had ''blown it'' and that his metabolism was ''shot,'' he worried that he would regain all his weight. In fact, Bill was ready to throw in the towel and start eating with abandon. That's exactly what he had done five years earlier, when the same rapid weight gain had occurred after a 120-pound weight loss.

I had great difficulty convincing Bill to remain patient. He couldn't quite believe that the weight gain he was experiencing was water and that he was still actually losing fat.

We kept Bill's calories at 1,300 but cut back on his carbohydrate choices to help him reduce fluid retention. Sure enough, the next week he *lost* 20 pounds. Heartened by this accomplishment, he joined a weight-maintenance support group, and now, eighteen months later, he continues to do well.

Note: This kind of increased fluid retention can occur with any weight-loss program, but it tends to be worse when the person is eating *high* G-Index foods. In part, the explanation lies in the way insulin acts on our body fat. Insulin, which is increased by high G-Index foods, acts directly on the kidneys to promote fluid retention. This is partly what happened with Bill, Laura, and many others.

Laura proceeded to shape her own G-Index Diet with favorite foods low on the Glycemic Index. For example, she included many fruits and also a considerable amount of low-fat and non-fat yogurt.

One simple dish she ate almost every day was old-fashioned oatmeal topped with skim milk and sweetened with one packet of fructose. For lunch, she usually had a cup of plain yogurt with wheat germ and fruit mixed in. She stayed away from pineapple, watermelon, and carrots because of her discouraging experience on the watermelon-pineapple diet. But she certainly could have eaten them in modest amounts, mixed with genuinely low GI foods. As for snacks, Laura included orange wedges and pears.

For her evening meal, she ate one moderate helping of various types of lean meat or fish, and she always piled on as many vegetables as possible, especially broccoli and asparagus. These and many other vegetables are relatively low on the Glycemic Index and quite consistent with the G-Index concept. When she didn't feel like cooking, she microwaved an entree from Healthy Choice, Weight Watchers, Lean Cuisine, or other makers of frozen diet entrees as the basis for her meal.

Fortunately, Laura knew from her many past dietary failures where her weaknesses lay. I've already mentioned her bad experiences with bread; she tended to stay away from it. Just in case she did feel the need for a piece, she kept a supply of coarse sprouted wheat or whole-grain European rye bread from the health food store in her cupboard.

She also discovered that dried fruits trigger her appetite. Raisins, dates, and the like are quite high on the Glycemic Index. So if Laura needed a sweetener, she usually sprinkled on a little table sugar.

With this program firmly established, Laura was able to continue to lose weight, and at her last evaluation, she was down to her second goal of 140. With the loss of this additional 30 pounds on the G-Index Diet, she was well on her way to avoiding the seesaw syndrome.

Why Exercise Is Also Important

There is every reason to believe that Laura will *continue* to lose weight, not only because she is firmly committed to the G-Index concept but because she has discovered exercise.

When she dropped to around 150, she found she had much more energy than she knew what to do with. Watching friends walking, jogging, and participating in various aerobics programs began to fascinate her. She wondered, "Would *I* be able to do that, when I've never exercised before in my life?"

To find out, Laura started a graduated aerobic walking program. Overcoming sore muscles and establishing a regular, new discipline gave her some second thoughts in the first few weeks. It took her a month and a half to reach a half-mile stretch at a time because she was feeling sore from muscles she had never really used before. But gradually she became stronger and more fit. Now she rises at 5:30 every morning and often walks briskly for more than an hour, four days a week.

Certainly the centerpiece of our program is the G-Index concept. But we've also found that long-term maintenance success depends on the number of miles a person walks. Regular exercise not only burns calories but also helps reinforce the diet by making a person feel good about herself and the way she looks. As a bonus, regular exercise reduces the body's tendency to overreact to sugar intake with blood sugar and insulin surges. In a very real sense, getting into shape turns down your G-Index thermostat and provides you with better tolerance for occasional high GI foods.

A final word on Laura and her comprehensive commitment to the G-Index concept: If I were a betting man, I'd place my money on her to conquer permanently a weight problem that began in childhood.

CHALLENGE 4:
A DIET TO COUNTER THE HIGH-STRESS BINGE

In most cases, people under stress eat more in order to counter the pressures and tensions in their lives. A person may turn to high-calorie, sweet, or fatty foods because these dishes are *pleasant* and they offer a temporary antidote to the stress.

This sort of stress-inspired binge diet is a dead-end street—for several reasons.

- Eating too much puts on excess pounds *and* adds a psychological component that escalates tension by making you feel worse about yourself. As your waistline grows larger, your self-confidence and sense of self-esteem plummet.
- The extra pounds you put on reduce the energy you have available to deal effectively with the pressures and stresses of life. The tension may arise primarily from work you haven't been able to finish. But if you don't have the get-up-and-go to get things done, the anxiety will increase.

- There is a physiologic reason for heightened rather than reduced stress when you overeat. You'll recall that foods high on the Glycemic Index—desserts, breads, and other goodies that often demolish diets—first tend to drive up blood sugar quickly. Then, the body releases a great surge of insulin, which causes the sugar to drop to low levels.
- At the bottom of this slide, the fight-or-flight hormone, adrenaline, rushes into the bloodstream to *stop* the downward direction of the blood sugar and to turn it back up. But when adrenaline enters the picture, a person becomes more edgy and tense. In other words, the high Glycemic Index food can actually increase the stress in your life!

To sum up, then, the G-Index Diet is an ideal counter to stress, anxiety, and tension because the diet increases your sense of self-esteem by helping you look trimmer; it increases your energy levels by keeping off extra weight; and it limits the release of adrenaline in your body, thus keeping you calmer through a better balance of your body chemistry.

How Frank Countered Stress with Food

Frank, a middle management executive, was constantly under pressure. He had two bosses who failed to coordinate their demands on him, and as a result, he sometimes felt he was holding down two jobs for the price of one. He had tried talking with each of these bosses individually, and both sympathized. But in the last analysis, they continued to put pressure on him because neither was willing to relieve Frank of any responsibilities.

The pressures also mounted in his family life. When he arrived home at night, often at a relatively late hour, his wife deluged him with questions and requests about household matters. And he rarely got to bed without engaging in an argument or delivering a lecture to his adolescent son or daughter.

Frank found that the only relief (and enjoyment) he could get during the day was to follow this routine:

- Have a cocktail before lunch.
- Eat high-fat sandwiches and beef dishes for his afternoon meal.
- Order a dessert after lunch.
- Have a brownie, chocolate bar, or cupcake as an afternoon snack.
- Drink eight to ten cups of coffee during the day.
- Polish off half a bag of potato chips or pretzels and a couple of mixed drinks when he arrived home in the evening.
- Consume several pieces of bread and at least one baked potato almost every night.
- Eat a dessert consisting of cake, pie, cookies, or some other sweet.
- Finish off the day with a big dish of ice cream or some other snack.

Needless to say, Frank's body began to show the results of this prodigious intake. He went from an ideal weight of 165 in his early twenties to a weight of 205 in his early forties. Furthermore, all this food didn't reduce his stress a bit. In fact, he felt more tense and anxious than ever before. The situation at work seemed to get worse, as did his home life.

Frank's blood pressure moved up to the hypertensive range, at 161/96 mmHg, and his personal physician recommended a rigorous weight-loss and exercise program in an attempt to bring that reading down. If these life-style changes didn't work, Frank was told, he would have to go on an antihypertensive medication.

To make matters worse, Frank's cholesterol crept up to 255 mm/dl, or 55 points higher than the recommended safe limit. His "bad" cholesterol (LDL, or low-density lipoprotein) was at 190, when it should have been below 130.

Frank seemed a prime candidate for a heart attack, particularly since his father had suffered one when he was barely fifty. Clearly, this man's diet wasn't working in the long run to reduce the stress in his life or to reduce the risks of cardiovascular disease.

On a brighter note, however, Frank was also a good candidate for improving his health by changing his diet and exercise habits. For most people, losing weight, increasing aerobic (or endurance) exercise, and limiting the intake of saturated fat and cholesterol in the diet will lower blood cholesterol and blood pressure.

I placed Frank on a G-Index Diet and suggested at the same time that he consider both starting an exercise program and trying some stress-reduction techniques.

- *The G-Index Solution*. I explained to Frank how his eating habits were contributing to his weight gain and to his stress level. He was fascinated to learn how the high Glycemic Index foods he was eating, such as the breads, pastries, and even baked (as opposed to boiled) potatoes, were sharpening his appetite. Also, he saw that his stress was increased by the release of adrenaline when his blood sugar plummeted.

  Next, I explained that his high consumption of coffee and alcohol were *also* increasing his hunger; various studies have established that caffeine and alcohol stimulate the appetite.

  Finally, we worked out a way for him to eat more foods he liked that were *low* on the Glycemic Index and to get rid of those that were high. For example, I had him substitute boiled potatoes (which have a moderate rating on the index) for his baked potatoes (high on the index).

- *The relaxation solution*. Frank sought help from a psychotherapist who was an expert in relaxation techniques. She had him spend ten to twenty minutes each day doing various mental exercises that calmed him down.

  For example, in some sessions, he listened to a tape with soothing, outdoor sounds. Also, he had some success with visualization techniques, which involved picturing a pleasant, peaceful scene in his mind and contemplating it for ten minutes or so.

- *The exercise solution*. Frank began to exercise again. He had been athletic in his youth, and as he lost weight, he found that his increased energy levels made him want to work out. So after a thorough checkup to be sure that he didn't have an underlying cardiovascular condition, he joined a tennis group and also started a walk-jog program. He pursued this regimen about four days a week.

The result of this change in life-style was dramatic. Frank's weight dropped from 205 to 165—his objective—in only four months. And he did it on his own through the G-Index Diet, without any need for liquid protein. Also, his blood cholesterol fell below 200, and his LDLs went below 130. At the same time, his increased athletic activity raised the level of his "good" cholesterol (HDL, or high-density lipoprotein).

As for his blood pressure, the readings are now down to a borderline level of 142/91. If Frank continues his progress, there is a good chance that he'll soon reach the normal range (below 140/90) without antihypertensive medication.

Perhaps most important of all, Frank was able to handle the pressure and tension in his life much more effectively. The physiological and emotional factors that had been triggering the stress have lost much of their power. Through a combination of the G-Index Diet, exercise, and relaxation techniques, Frank has completely changed his life.

Such experiences are being repeated every day among those who are discovering the many benefits of the G-Index Diet. To be sure, there are some problems—such as certain deep-rooted emotional disturbances or overwhelming food cravings—that are impervious to any diet. These require special medical or psychological attention. But *most* people, with *most* dietary concerns, can find the answer to weight loss and also end the seesaw syndrome with the G-Index approach.

Now let's turn to a more specific description of the diet and some principles and tactics that will allow you to make the best use of it.

CHAPTER THREE

The Basics of the G-Index Diet

The G-Index Diet is based on several simple principles that have been firmly established in scientific and medical research. Specifically, the diet has been designed with the following food plan in mind:

- Specially selected sugars and carbohydrates that prevent wild swings in blood sugar and insulin—*and* in appetite.
- Low amounts of fat, especially saturated fat. *Note:* Each day's menus in this book contain only about 25 percent of calories from fats, and saturated fats are always less than one-third of total fat calories.
- High amounts of fiber.
- Low to moderate calorie intake.
- *No* "forbidden" foods. *Anything* can be eaten, so long as certain basic ground rules are observed.

What is so distinctive about the foods and eating tactics in the G-Index Diet? To introduce you to the ways that this diet differs from others, I've formulated a comparison of the G-Index approach to a standard American diet and a typical low-calorie diet.

HOW THE G-INDEX DIET IS DIFFERENT

In the following summaries, typical foods are compared in three types of diets for breakfast, lunch, dinner, and snack time.

The first diet is a standard American diet, which pays no particular attention to low-fat or high-fiber foods, and reflects typical American eating habits.

The second diet is a typical low-fat, high-fiber, high Glycemic Index diet, similar to what many weight-reduction programs use. This diet is low in calories but will not help you control your appetite.

The third diet is a low-fat, high-fiber, low GI diet consistent with the G-Index Diet. This approach will help you control your appetite through better regulation of your blood sugar and insulin.

Breakfast

Standard American Diet: Corn flakes (sugar added) with whole milk and sugar; white toast with butter; 2 pieces of bacon; orange juice; coffee.

Most Diet Programs: Oat bran flakes (honey added) with skim milk and raisins; whole wheat toast with diet margarine; orange juice; coffee.

G-Index Diet: Old-fashioned oatmeal, All-Bran, or Fiber One cereal (fructose added as sweetener); pear slices; whole-grain toast with diet margarine; 1 small slice of drained bacon; orange juice; coffee.

Lunch

Standard American Diet: Ham and cheese sandwich on white bread with mayonnaise; potato chips; carbonated soft drink.

Most Diet Programs: Turkey (white meat) sandwich on regular whole wheat bread with reduced calorie mayonnaise; lettuce and tomato salad with low-calorie dressing; diet soda.

G-Index Diet: Turkey (white meat) sandwich on 100 percent sprouted, cracked wheat, or stone-ground whole wheat bread with reduced calorie mayonnaise; pasta, bean, and chickpea salad with low-calorie dressing; skim milk.

Dinner

Standard American Diet: Dinner roll and butter; fried chicken; french fries; tomato and lettuce salad with creamy dressing; ice cream.

Most Diet Programs: Commercial high-fiber muffin; broiled chicken breast; baked potato; carrots; lima beans; sugar-sweetened low-fat frozen yogurt.

G-Index Diet: Mixed green salad (asparagus, spinach, radishes, string beans, pinto beans); broiled chicken breast; boiled potato; broccoli; low-calorie salad dressing; fresh strawberries; 1 small square of chocolate or 1 small piece of cheese or sugar-free low-fat frozen yogurt.

Snack

Standard American Diet: Doughnut, or commercial chocolate-chip cookies; soda.

Most Diet Programs: Pineapple juice; raisins; high-fiber muffin (primarily flour-based, with fiber added).

G-Index Diet: Toasted pita bread or high-fiber muffin (fruit-based—e.g., Muffin-a-Day or R. W. Frookie cookies); 1 one-inch square cheddar cheese; frozen yogurt cup (no sugar added); orange juice.

The first diet—the Standard American diet—has relatively high quantities of fat, especially the saturated kind. So this approach doesn't fit the current medical recommendations for a low-fat, low-cholesterol program, which is necessary to keep the risk of cardiovascular disease, cancer, and other ills as low as possible. Also, as you'll see in the next chapter, many of the foods on this diet, such as the dinner roll and cookies, are high on the Glycemic Index and thus trigger hunger.

The second diet—most diet programs—eliminates the fat but not the *hunger*. Many of the foods listed, though high in fiber and generally nutritious, contain carbohydrates with a high Glycemic Index: baked potatoes, most commercial whole wheat bread, carrots, lima beans, and the primarily flour-based muffin. Consequently, dieters who eat these foods tend to become hungry within a couple of hours after a meal.

The third diet—G-Index plan—has all the health benefits of the second but it avoids hunger-triggering foods that are high on the Glycemic Index. Consequently, this diet enables someone to take weight off and keep it off.

Furthermore, the G-Index approach includes no "forbidden" foods—just guidelines about how much of certain foods should be eaten to succeed at weight loss. For example, one slice of bacon is included in the breakfast, a small square of cheese as a snack, and a small square of chocolate with the evening meal. With most diets, these foods are "no-no's"—they contain too much saturated fat and thus add too many calories, not to mention that they endanger the cardiovascular system.

But with the G-Index Diet, some "bad," fatty foods may be recommended *in small quantities* as a prescriptive means of holding off hunger. Fat acts much like carbohydrates that are low on the Glycemic Index, in that it feeds slowly through the digestive system and into the blood, thus moderating the movement of blood sugar and insulin. It's better to eat a little fat and keep your appetite under control, than to eat none and go on a binge that breaks your diet.

Caution: Some people with serious cholesterol or other blood lipid (fat) problems may be directed by their physicians to stay away from even these small, prescriptive amounts of fat. Others who have particular food cravings may find that they can't eat a little of these foods without gorging themselves.

If you're in either of these categories, you may have to modify the fat prescription concept. Fortunately, many healthy foods contain unsaturated fats that do not raise cholesterol. For example, all these provide a relatively low 45 calories and 5 grams of fat: 6 almonds, 10 unsalted large peanuts, 2 teaspoons of pumpkin seeds; 5 large olives, 2 tablespoons of guacamole mix; and one teaspoon of vegetable oil on a salad. Of course, to accommodate these fats, you'll have to monitor your fat intake throughout the day.

Now, with this overview of the G-Index Diet in mind, let's consider how the foods in the G-Index Diet are ranked.

UNDERSTANDING THE G-INDEX FOOD RANKING SYSTEM

As you now know, low GI foods are intended to provide a slow, steady input of sugar into the blood to avoid disruptive surges of blood sugar and insulin, which can trigger hunger. The wrong carbohydrates can also alter the body's metabolism by reducing your ability to burn calories, a process that will increase your storage of fat.

The original Glycemic Index, as devised and used by researchers investigating diabetes, ranges from the low double-digit numbers for low GI foods to triple-digit numbers for very high GI foods. For example, white or regular whole wheat bread is given a 100 rating, which is quite high on the index. In contrast, spaghetti and other pastas get a relatively low 66. A pear is a low 47; a grapefruit receives a 36; and a plum is 34.

HOW THE G-INDEX RATINGS ARE DETERMINED

To determine the G-Index of a food, fasting volunteers eat several meals, each containing a prescribed amount of a single test-food. Portions are adjusted so that each meal contains the same amount of carbohydrate, usually 50 grams, which is roughly 1.5 ounces. Blood sugar (glucose) levels are measured before and after eating over the course of the next several hours. The G-Index is calculated based on the rise and duration of blood sugar elevation—what mathematicians call the "area under the curve." The rise and duration of blood sugar elevation for each test food is compared with the rise and duration for a "standard" food, usually white bread. The standard food is arbitrarily assigned a G-Index of 100.

Thus, foods such as most fruits, which do not produce a high or long rise in blood sugar, have a G-Index rating below 100 (typically 40–60). Foods such as baked potatoes, honey, or oat bran flakes, which produce a rise in blood glucose that is higher or longer than white bread, have a score over 100.

Slow digestion tends to produce a low (desirable) G-Index. Properties of a food which slow the pace of digestion include compactness rather than crumbliness (pasta rather than bread); sturdy resistance to digestive enzyme (less refined whole grain rather than moderately refined wholemeal); and high fiber rather than low fiber.

In addition to a slow speed of digestion, a low G-Index will occur if the food contains mainly those forms of carbohydrate which do not biochemically convert into glucose, such as fructose (fruit sugar). That's why orange juice, for example, has a low G-Index despite its lack of fiber and rapid digestion.

SIMPLIFYING THE SYSTEM FOR DIETERS

To make it easier to identify and select foods with a low Glycemic Index, and to avoid those with a high GI, I've reclassified a wide variety of foods into four categories. (For an extensive listing, see the G-Index exchange lists in Chapter Eight.) Foods that are in the first (1) and second (2) categories are low on the Glycemic Index and should be preferred by all dieters. Pears, grapefruit, and plums are all rated 1. These items are always more filling, have the power to cut hunger, and are often more nutritious than high GI foods.

Those foods in the third category (3) are moderately desirable for the diet. Examples are boiled potatoes, corn, bananas, and table sugar (sucrose). Those in the fourth group (4) are less desirable, in that they lead to quick and sharp rises in blood sugar and insulin, and a greater appetite. White and whole wheat bread and baked or instant potatoes are in class 4.

Note: Technically, fats can't be rated according to the Glycemic Index—only carbohydrates qualify for this scale. But fats *do* affect blood sugar and insulin in that they cause them to rise slowly, much like a low GI carbohydrate. Consequently, I've broadened the Glycemic Index concept a bit and given a favorable, low rating (usually a 1*) to fats, *but with this caveat:* Any fats that are consumed must be eaten in *very* small quantities—no more than the amounts indicated in the various lists, menus, or recipes. To remind you of the special status of fats, whenever their ratings are listed the number is followed by an asterisk (*).

Also, remember that any fats you consume are to be used prescriptively. Usually, this means eating them in small quantities at the end of a meal or at other times during the day to help ward off hunger.

Finally, I've allowed some "cheating" on the diet by including occasional foods in categories 3 or even 4. I know that practically everyone on a diet nibbles occasionally on things they know they "shouldn't" eat. The secret to dieting success is usually not to avoid these foods completely but, rather, to eat them in quantities and at times that won't break the basic weight-loss program. In any event, category 3 and especially 4 foods must be carefully limited. Otherwise, they will trigger the appetite, the seesaw phenomenon will be set in motion, and the pounds will return.

Now, with these basics in mind, let's move on to a more detailed consideration of how you can identify the various foods that suppress hunger. This information will both make it easier for you to use the menus and recipes that we've prepared, and also give you a solid foundation to build your *individual* food plan through the food exchange system described in Chapter Eight.

CHAPTER FOUR

A Guide to the Foods That Suppress Hunger

To make the best use of the G-Index Diet, it's essential that you have a firm grasp of the various types of foods that suppress appetite, and also those that trigger hunger.

To equip you for this task, I've highlighted the G-Index status of many common foods likely to end up on your table. The discussion of each food has been capped by ratings of the foods under three headings:

- Low GI (highly desirable)
- Intermediate GI (moderately desirable)
- High GI (less desirable)

Low GI foods include those with a 1 or 2 rating, as discussed in the previous chapter. Intermediate GI foods have a 3 rating; and high GI foods have a 4 rating. Most of your foods on this diet should come from the low GI category, or have a *1* or *2* rating. But it's quite all right to mix in some intermediate and even high GI foods, so long as they are balanced by those with a low Glycemic Index.

To provide you with a handy overview of how certain Key Foods are categorized on the diet, see the accompanying "G-Index Diet At A Glance." The details follow.

G-INDEX DIET AT A GLANCE

DESIRABLE FOODS	MODERATELY DESIRABLE FOODS	LESS DESIRABLE FOODS
Breads:		
Coarse European-Style Whole Grain Wheat or Rye Pita Bread Cracked or Sprouted Whole Wheat Bread	100% Stone Ground Whole Wheat Pumpernickel 100% Whole Stoneground Whole Wheat Matzoh 100% Whole Grain Rye Crisp crackers	White bread Most commercial whole wheat breads Most commercial North American Rye Bread English Muffin, Bagel, Most Commercial Matzoh
Cereals:		
Compact noodle-like high bran cereals, e.g., All-Bran, Fiber One Coarse Oatmeal Porridge Coarse Whole Grain Cereal, e.g., Kashi Breakfast Pilaf Cereal mixed with Psyllium, e.g., Fiberwise	Grape-nut Cereal Medium/fine grain Oatmeal Porridge, e.g., "5 Minute" variety	Flaked Cereals Puffed Cereals Instant, "Quick" or Pre-cooked Cereals

DESIRABLE FOODS	MODERATELY DESIRABLE FOODS	LESS DESIRABLE FOODS
Pastas, Grains, and Starchy Vegetables: Pasta (all types) Barley, Bulgur, Buckwheat (Kasha), Couscous Most Beans and Peas Sweet Potato, Yam	Rice Boiled Potato Corn	Instant, "Quick" or Precooked Grains Baked Potato Lima Beans Winter Squash (acorn, butternut)
Milk Products: Skim Milk; 1% Milk, all cottage cheese (low fat or regular) Buttermilk Low-fat Plain Yogurt Low-fat fruited Yogurt with artificial sweetener Low-fat artificially sweetened desserts, e.g., Creamsicle Low-fat frozen Yogurt with artificial sweetener	2% Milk Cheese Regular Plain Yogurt Simple Pleasures	Whole Milk, Ice Milk, Ice Cream Yogurt sweetened with sugar (including low-fat varieties) Low-fat frozen desserts with sugar added Low-fat and regular frozen yogurt with sugar added

DESIRABLE FOODS	**MODERATELY DESIRABLE FOODS**	**LESS DESIRABLE FOODS**
Fruit:		
Most fruit and natural fruit juices including apple, berries, cantaloupe, grapefruit, honeydew, orange	Banana Kiwi Mango	Pineapple Raisin Watermelon Fruit juices sweetened with sugar
Vegetables:		
Almost all vegetables	Beets	Carrots Winter Squash (acorn, butternut)
Meat/Protein Foods (in Moderation):		
Shellfish "White" (Low-fat) fish, e.g., cod, flounder, trout, tuna in water Egg substitutes (cholesterol-free) Cottage Cheese Venison Chicken, turkey, cornish hen (white meat/no skin)	Higher fat fish, e.g., Salmon, Herring Lean cuts of Beef, Pork, Veal Low-fat "imitation" luncheon meat Low-fat cheese Egg	Most cuts of beef, pork, lamb Hot dog (including "low-fat" versions) Cheese Luncheon Meat Peanut butter, Peanuts (take only in the strictly limited amounts prescribed in diet plan)

DESIRABLE FOODS	MODERATELY DESIRABLE FOODS	LESS DESIRABLE FOODS
Fats: Take only in strictly limited amounts prescribed in diet to attain 25% calories from fat. Emphasize vegetable oil and seafood sources low in saturated fat		Meat and dairy derived fat, high in saturated fat
Soups: Low-fat, low G-Index versions, e.g., Health Valley, Nile Spice, Pritikin, Progresso (certain varieties, e.g., Vegetable), Campbell Healthy Request Brands (certain varieties, e.g., Chicken Noodle, Minestrone)	Most commercial soups contain substantial fat, high-G-Index starch added or both as well as high salt.	Powdered ''Cup-of Soup''-type instant soups usually contain corn syrup

DESIRABLE FOODS	MODERATELY DESIRABLE FOODS	LESS DESIRABLE FOODS
"Free" Foods:		
Bouillon, broth (low salt) Cocoa Powder		
Cabbage, Celery, Lettuce, Mushroom, Pickles, Radishes, Zucchini		
Gelatin (sugar-free), jams/jelly (sugar-free)		
Catsup, Mustard, Salad Dressing (very low calorie varieties)		
Sugars:		
Take only in strictly limited amounts	Artificial sweeteners, e.g., Equal	Glucose Corn syrup Honey Molasses
Fructose	Artificially sweetened, non-caffeinated soda	Sucrose (in more than strictly limited amounts)
Lactose	Sucrose (in strictly limited amounts)	
	Artificially sweetened desserts	

THE G-INDEX STRATEGY STARTS WITH THE STARCHES

Starch foods consist mainly of carbohydrates, have a modest amount of protein, and have almost no fat. The main starches include breads and crackers; cereal, grains, and pasta; beans, peas, and lentils; and starchy vegetables.

Starches, especially breads and cereals, are mostly high GI foods that trigger the blood sugar and insulin surges that control our appetites. So choose your starch foods wisely for success on the G-Index Diet.

Breads

Most breads and cereals cause a more rapid and higher blood sugar rise than an equal amount of most other carbohydrate foods. Because bread crumbles easily into many tiny particles, the starch is thoroughly exposed to the digestive enzymes of the stomach and small intestine. Digestion converts starch almost instantly into glucose molecules, which are rapidly absorbed into the blood and elevate the blood sugar level.

How can you identify the best breads for your diet? First, whole wheat and white bread—regardless of their differences in nutritional value—are equally bad for appetite suppression. Whole wheat bread flour has received somewhat less processing than white bread flour, but the processing of most whole wheat flour is still extensive enough to cause rapid digestion and a high Glycemic Index. The same holds true for most commercial, North American rye breads. Breads that are milled less completely—such as 100 percent stone-ground whole wheat, and pumpernickel rye—have moderate G-Index values of about 3. Some moderately low G-Index stone-ground whole wheat breads include Arnold Stone-ground 100% Whole Wheat Bread and Pepperidge Farm Sprouted Wheat Bread.

The only breads that have excellent, low GI levels (a rating of 1 or 2) are those of the coarse, predominantly whole-grain, sprouted, or cracked wheat variety, or European-style rye breads. The minimally processed particles in these breads, which are similar to what Americans ate in the early 1700s, digest more slowly than standard breads.

Although most commercial whole meal or whole wheat breads are less refined than white breads, they are still more highly processed—and thus, more rapidly digested—than are breads made from whole grains. Sprouted and cracked grains are refined relatively little, though they are more refined than whole grain. Stone ground whole wheat is more refined than sprouted or cracked wheat, but less so than other wholemeal or whole wheat breads.

But don't be misled by labels! Many commercial rye breads are made from highly processed flour with molasses or caramel added as a darkener. A bread labeled "sprouted wheat" might actually contain refined wheat flour, corn syrup, and vegetable oil as its main components, with just a little sprouted wheat thrown in to "dress up" the label. *Note:* Ingredients on labels are listed in order of their descending quantity in the product. The Food and Drug Administration (FDA) regulates the formal food label but does not closely monitor what could be considered misleading claims elsewhere on the wrapping.

One subjective way to determine whether a bread is high or low on the Glycemic Index is whether it melts in your mouth. If it does, you probably have a high GI food; if it doesn't, the food most likely has a low GI. True low G-Index coarse wheat or European-style rye breads are only occasionally found in supermarkets or commercial bakeries. More often, you must buy them in health food stores. Many are local rather than "national" brands.

More specifically, the G-Index bread ratings are as follows:

- *Low GI (highly desirable):* European-style coarse rye bread; wheat breads made from predominantly whole grain, sprouted or cracked wheat, such as Shiloh Farms 100 Percent Whole Grain and sprouted Wheat Bread; Ezekiel 4:9 Sprouted Grain Bread; Vermont Bread Company's 100% Whole Grain Rye Bread, or 100% Stoneground Whole Wheat Bread; Wild's Whole Grain Bread; Alvarado Farms Sprouted Wheat Bagel; pita bread.

- *Intermediate GI (moderately desirable):* Stone-ground whole wheat bread, such as Arnold's Stoneground 100% Whole Wheat Bread, Matthew's All Natural Whole Wheat Bread, or Pepperidge Farm Stone Ground 100% Whole Wheat Bread; Orowheat Whole Wheat Bread; pumpernickel bread; 100% whole grain rye crisp crackers (Ry Krisp, Wasa); 100% stone ground whole wheat matzoh; Brownberry Breads (Natural Wheat, Natural 12 Grain, Natural Rye, Natural Health Nut); Jewel Company Bread (7 Grain, Oat Bran).
- *High GI (less desirable):* Most whole wheat bread; commercial rye bread, white bread, wheat crackers, English muffins, bread sticks, regular matzoh, pretzels, commercial bagel.

(See also pages 192 and 281 for more information about breads.)

Cereals

Most breakfast cereals have a GI rating similar to white bread. Old-fashioned oatmeal and cooked oat bran have a somewhat lower GI, particularly if relatively coarse. But when oat bran is pounded into cereal flakes or produced in "instant" hot cereal form, its integrity is disrupted and its Glycemic Index is raised.

Note: Oat bran flakes may have just as much fiber as hot oatmeal porridge cereal, but the GI of oat bran flakes is 20 percent higher than that of white bread! In contrast, the GI of oatmeal porridge is 20 percent lower than that of white bread. These products may be nutritionally comparable in most respects, but for weight-loss purposes the hot cereal is superior.

Similarly, "puffing" a cereal, even a whole-grain cereal, accelerates digestion and increases the Glycemic Index. Kashi Breakfast Pilaf, for instance, has a relatively low G-Index rating, but Puffed Kashi has a high one.

All-Bran, Fiber One, and other "spaghetti-shaped" cereals have a relatively low G-Index. I suspect that their shape, rather than their high bran content, is the reason, since most other high-bran cereals with different shapes have a high GI.

Kellogg has come up with an interesting way to reduce the GI of a high GI cereal: mix it thoroughly with a very low GI fiber. Fiberwise (formerly called Heartwise) contains whole wheat and oat bran flakes mixed with psyllium, a very low GI fiber. (Psyllium, by the way, is a component of anticonstipation medicines such as Metamucil.)

Mixed with psyllium, the Fiberwise cereal has a relatively low GI, since psyllium slows the passage of the meal through the stomach and retards digestion of the cereal.

Actually, you could get the same G-Index lowering effect by mixing psyllium with your favorite cereal. Usually, though, this do-it-yourself approach tastes terrible. Kellogg's version masks the undesirable psyllium taste.

Here are the G-Index cereal ratings (see also cereal lists on pages 190 and 280):

- *Low GI (highly desirable).* Kellogg's All-Bran (preferably sugar-free) and General Mills Fiber One or other "spaghetti-shaped" bran cereals; Kellogg's Fiberwise; old-fashioned oatmeal; whole-grain cereal (not puffed) such as Kashi Breakfast Pilaf.
- *Intermediate GI (moderately desirable).* Post Grape-Nuts; fine-grain oatmeal (such as the five-minute type).
- *High GI (less desirable).* Flaked cereals, including oat bran, corn flakes, or others; puffed cereals, including Kashi; most processed, ready-to-eat cereals such as muesli, shredded wheat, or Weetabix; instant, quick, or precooked cereals such as instant or one-minute oatmeal.

Pasta and Other Grains

Pasta of all types has a low GI, whether it's made from whole wheat or white flour. Pasta raises the blood sugar only about two-thirds as much as the same number of calories of bread.

Why the difference? Pasta pieces are large and compact. The digestive enzymes have to start at the surface and work their way slowly through the product. It's true that all the carbohydrate in pasta eventually converts into glucose, but the process takes much longer than with bread.

The lesson for dieters is that, calorie for calorie, pasta suppresses the appetite longer and promotes fat-burning better than the same number of calories eaten as bread.

Rice has a moderate G-Index rating—not as good as pasta but better than most breads and cereals. But different studies report a fairly wide range of values for rice, a fact suggesting that different strains, or different cooking methods, give different results. The more nutritious brown rice has no G-Index advantage over the highly refined and less nutritious white variety. More research is needed for us to make a definitive judgment on rice. For now, it's best to assume a medium G-Index rating for both white and brown rice.

Other grains have been established as superior hunger-suppressors. For example, barley, bulgur (cracked wheat), and buckwheat (actually a fruit) as found in kasha are low on the GI scale. Some newer health-food grains such as amaranth have yet to be tested for their G-Index effect.

Here are the G-Index grain and pasta ratings:

- *Low GI (highly desirable).* Buckwheat (kasha), barley, bulgur, couscous, pasta (all types).
- *Intermediate GI (moderately desirable).* White or brown rice.
- *High GI (less desirable).* Instant, "quick," or precooked grains; millet.

Muffins, Crackers, and Snacks

Most crackers or muffins are either high in fat or high on the G-Index. There are exceptions, however. For example, the Apples 'n' Oats Muffin recipe on page 136 has a low GI.

My favorite commercial muffin, Muffin-A-Day, has a low GI but isn't yet available in some places. You can order it, however, by telephone from anywhere in the country by calling 1-800-258-8961. This product contains no fat and uses a tasty mix of fruit fibers to replace most of the high G-Index wheat flour that would otherwise be the primary ingredient.

Surprisingly, graham crackers tested out quite well on the GI scale, with a rating of 2. Perhaps the modest fat content in these cookies slows down its digestion.

Cookies sweetened largely with fructose (fruit sugar), such as from R. W. Frookie, have a reasonably low Glycemic Index. These can be found in the diet food or diabetes food section of the supermarket and in most health food stores.

Popcorn is a GI disappointment. We tested a light-version air-popped popcorn and found it to have a high G-Index, so popcorn should not be considered an appetite-suppressing snack. In fact, eating more than a small amount of popcorn tends to *increase* your appetite within a few hours.

Note: G-Index evaluations compare food portions that contain equal quantities of carbohydrate calories—200 calories, to be exact. That means that about eight cups of popcorn have to be used for the test. Obviously, this is a large amount for one person to consume. Eating one cup of popcorn would raise the blood sugar only a little and wouldn't cause a large insulin rebound. Small amounts of high GI foods like popcorn won't help you diet, but they won't destroy it, either. Large amounts *are* a problem, however. The goal of a snack is to provide a slow, steady blood sugar flow for several hours, without a sharp rise that sets off an insulin surge. Popcorn doesn't provide this benefit.

Similar considerations apply to rice crackers. Although they have only about 35 calories each, their relatively high GI rating requires that they be eaten in small amounts. If you put some fruited jelly with a low GI on them, however, a snack of one rice cracker can make sense.

Most presweetened commercial yogurts, including regular and frozen, are considered starches for nutritional purposes rather than dairy products, since high quantities of sugar are added and, consequently, they have a lower proportion of protein than would be expected for milk products. Because most producers use high G-Index sugars, these are usually high GI foods. Fortunately, there are some exceptions, including low-fat plain yogurt, fruited yogurt with artificial sweeteners instead of sugar, and frozen yogurt with artificial sweeteners. All these have an excellent, low G-Index.

Here are the G-Index ratings for muffins, crackers, and snacks (see also snack food lists, pages 260 and 282):

- *Low GI (highly desirable).* Fruit-based muffins such as on page 136, Muffin-A-Day muffins, and Health Valley Fat-Free Apple Spice Muffins; Ak-Mak 100% stone ground whole wheat cracker; cookies such as Health Valley Fat-Free Date Delight Cookies, Health Valley Fat-Free Apple-Fruit Bars, Nature's Choice Oat Bran Bars, Nature's Choice Real Fruit Bar; fructose-based cookies such as R. W. Frookie; nonfat, artificially flavored frozen yogurt, nonfat, fruited, artificially flavored yogurt, and plain yogurt (also see milk list for other yogurt choices). *Note:* Ultra Slim-Fast commercial food supplement (essentially flavored skim milk, highly sweetened with fructose) has a favorable G-Index rating.
- *Intermediate GI (moderately desirable).* Graham crackers, Fig Newtons, Fifty Chocolate Chip Diabetic Cookies.
- *High GI (less desirable).* Popcorn, puffed rice cakes, potato chips, pretzels, most commercial muffins and cookies, nonfat yogurt with added sugar, nonfat frozen yogurt with added sugar.

Legumes (Beans, Peas) and Starchy Vegetables

Although Americans depend heavily on cereal grains, we tend to *underuse* the starchy legumes.

Beans are extremely high in fiber, particularly cholesterol-lowering water-soluble fiber. Also, they are quite filling. Their vitamin and mineral content is superior to that of highly processed grains, and they are relatively high in protein. In fact, legume family members—such as soybean, kidney bean, lentil and chickpea—are classed by nutritionists as a meat rather than a starch because of their high protein content.

The main problem with beans is that, like all other high-fiber foods, they tend to cause gas. Fiber is only partly digested by the human digestive enzymes in the upper part of the gastrointestinal tract. But when the food reaches the large intestine, or colon, the bacteria there begin to break it down. That process causes gas.

The appearance of gas is most striking when you switch abruptly from a low- to a high-fiber diet. It's less of a problem when you add fiber little by little to your daily menus. But regardless of the amount of gas you experience, its production tends to decrease after about two months. You can reduce the gas in canned beans quite simply. Remove the water in which the beans have been soaking in the can. Then rinse the beans thoroughly.

Also, the way you cook beans can help reduce their gas-producing potential. Here are some guidelines:

1. Soak the beans for four to five hours, or overnight. Nine cups of water should be used for one cup of beans.
2. Discard the water you used for soaking and replace with the same amount of fresh water.
3. Cook beans for 30 minutes. Discard the water.
4. Add the same amount of water again, and cook the beans until they are soft.

An alternative preparation is to add baking soda to the soaking water. This helps leach out sugars, but also eliminates the thiamine (vitamin B_1).

Here's another possibility for gas reduction. A new digestive enzyme called Beano Drops is available without a prescription in many drug stores and health food stores. Taken just before eating, Beano Drops supply enzymes that help digest bean fiber, thus reducing its gas potential.

Here are some hints to help cut down on gas through the way you eat your meals:

1. Eat small amounts of beans at the beginning of your diet.
2. Don't mix beans with other gas-producing vegetables such as cabbage.

3. Don't undercook the beans; they should mash easily. Otherwise, the undercooked starch in them can cause gas.
4. Use low GI beans that produce the least amount of gas, including lentils and chickpeas.
5. For canned beans: remove the water in which the beans have been soaking in the can. Then rinse the beans thoroughly.

The potato is a starchy vegetable that is a major carbohydrate source for many Americans. Potatoes are a class 3 GI food when boiled, but baked potatoes are a high class 4. In fact, they have a GI one-third higher than white bread! So boil your potatoes, don't bake them.

Under no circumstances should you have a baked potato as a mid-afternoon snack. Although you could do much worse in terms of calories, baked potatoes have such a high GI that they cause significant insulin secretion. The result is greatly increased hunger before your next meal.

Note: A modest topping of sour cream or cheese—less than an ounce—will reduce the GI of a baked potato by slowing down its passage through the stomach. With careful diet planning, you could allocate a share of your daily fat quota for this topping and still maintain an overall low-fat regimen. Here, again, you see how the prescriptive use of fat can protect you against surges of high blood sugar and insulin.

Sweet potatoes or yams are lower on the GI scale and thus should be preferred over white potatoes.

Lima beans have a very high GI rating of 4. Unlike most other legumes, limas are thus undesirable for people who want to maintain their diets.

Corn kernels have an intermediate GI rating of 3. In other words, they may be eaten in moderate quantities by dieters. (Popped corn is much worse, probably because of the popping process.)

Here are the GI ratings of legumes and starchy vegetables:

- *Low GI (highly desirable).* Butter beans, chickpeas, cluster beans (guar gum), haricot beans, lentils, kidney beans, peas, pinto beans, soy beans, sweet potato or yam.

- *Intermediate GI (moderately desirable)*. Boiled potato, corn kernels.
- *High GI (less desirable)*. Lima beans; baked potato, instant potato, mashed potato, french fried potato, potato chips; winter squash (butternut, acorn).

IS THERE A SPOT IN YOUR DIET FOR SWEETENERS?

Most nutrition and diet books don't discuss sweeteners, at least not in positive terms, because these simple sugars are for the most part "empty calories." That is, they are nearly devoid of vitamins, minerals, and protein.

Still, when used appropriately, sweeteners can add to the pleasure of eating—and can actually be used to further a successful diet strategy. The secret to the wise use of sweeteners is to select them with an eye to their different Glycemic Index ratings.

Sugar has a reputation for triggering "hypoglycemic reactions," or sudden surges and plunges in blood sugar. This bad press is based largely on the disruptive effect of high G-Index sugars, such as corn syrup, honey, or glucose sweeteners.

In contrast, sugars such as fructose can actually *help* you with your diet. Both fructose (fruit sugar) and lactose (milk sugar) have a very low G-Index. As a result, when used in moderation, they can suppress the appetite. *Caution:* Diabetics who are at poor levels of blood sugar control often find that fructose raises their blood sugar almost as much as do glucose and other high G-Index sugars.

Interestingly, table sugar (sucrose), though not at the top of my list as a diet food, has a lower G-Index rating than white bread. Still, there are some significant problems with sucrose.

- Manufacturers hide enormous quantities of sucrose in their products. For example, a twelve-ounce soda might contain ten teaspoons of sugar, compared with five teaspoons in the entire blood volume of a typical adult!

- Many people find sugar addictive. The more they eat, the more they want—and the more they must consume before they can find that sweet taste again.

Still, one or two teaspoons a day of table sugar for your cereal or hot drink should do no harm. And by increasing your satisfaction with your food, these small amounts can actually help you maintain your diet.

Here are the GI ratings for sweeteners:

- *Low GI (highly desirable)*. Fructose, lactose, fruit jam or jelly with *only* fructose added.
- *Intermediate GI (moderately desirable)*. Sucrose, including table sugar and brown sugar.
- *High GI (less desirable)*. Corn syrup or sweetener, glucose, honey, molasses, maltose, commercial jams or jellies with sweetener added, maple syrup.

A note on artificial sweeteners: Like most nutritionists, I have mixed feelings about artificial, noncaloric sweeteners. On the positive side, they save considerable calories, and by themselves, they don't create blood sugar and insulin surges.

On the other hand, consuming large amounts of any kind of sweetened food or drink perpetuates the desire for sweets. Abstaining from sweets, both artificial and natural, reduces that desire after several weeks—a major blessing for dieters.

Another problem with artificial sweeteners is that they often are combined with caffeine or with high G-Index flours. For example, caffeine may be found in many cola drinks. High G-Index wheat flours are a major component of "diet" cookies. These foods promote blood sugar and insulin surges and can undermine your diet.

Here's the bottom line: You are much better off keeping sweets of all types to a minimum; after a while you will come to like it that way. But I have no serious objection to the use of moderate amounts of an artificial sweetener on cereal in the morning, in decaffeinated coffee, or as part of an occasional noncaffeinated diet soda.

The unusual person may develop headaches or experience

allergic reactions to these substances. But most scientists believe that artificial sweeteners currently in use are usually safe when taken in normal, modest amounts.

THE FANTASTIC DIET POTENTIAL OF FRUITS

Fruit consists of carbohydrates only, with essentially no protein or fat. Most important for our purposes, most fruits contain *fructose*, which is the most desirable diet sugar. Fructose is a great hunger-averter because it's a *low* class 1 on the GI scale; furthermore, ounce for ounce, fructose tastes much sweeter than table sugar.

Because the GI rating of fructose is so low, the GI of most fruits stays in the 1 or 2 categories. As a result, fruits are ideal between-meal snacks or as sweeteners to be added to cereal or plain yogurt. Grapefruit, cherries, plums, and pears are among the best diet foods for this purpose.

Fruit juices, despite their relative lack of fiber, have about the same GI as whole fruit. Still, whole fruit should remain the dieter's choice, in part because it takes more "work" to chew. It's easy to drink more juice than you intend because you can just gulp it down quickly. Also, whole fruit contains more fiber, and is more filling than juice.

Only a few fruits need to be approached with caution. The most important is the banana. Typically, bananas rate as moderate G-Index food (category 3)—much better than most sugars or bread, but not as low as other fruit. You might use the banana as a sweetener on your cereal or as a snack, but try to mix it with some lower G-Index fruit.

For example, you might combine half a banana with an apple half in your cereal or plain yogurt. Use the other half of each fruit later for a snack. Surprisingly, recent research has revealed that the G-Index for a ripe banana as opposed to new one is not much different.

Several other tropical fruits such as watermelon and pineapple are relatively high GI foods. Fortunately, cantaloupe and honeydew melon each have a relatively low GI.

Dried fruits are also a problem for dieters. Although grapes and plums have a low GI, their dried forms—raisins and prunes—are high GI foods. From a dieter's perspective, eating raisins is like eating white bread.

If you choose your fruit wisely—eating as much fruit as you can instead of fats or starches—you'll have a good prescription for dietary success.

Here are the GI ratings for fruit:

- *Low GI (highly desirable)*. Apples, applesauce, apricots, blackberries, blueberries, cantaloupe, cherries, honeydew melon, grapefruit, grapes, oranges, peaches, pears, plums, raspberries, strawberries, tangerines; fruit juices including unsweetened apple juice or cider, cranberry juice (diet version), grapefruit juice, grape juice, orange juice.
- *Intermediate GI (moderately desirable)*. Banana, kiwi, mango, papaya.
- *High GI (less desirable)*. Watermelon, prunes, prune juice, raisins, pineapple, sweetened fruit juice.

EAT YOUR VEGETABLES!

With very few exceptions, green, leafy vegetables are excellent, low GI foods. They are also high in vitamins, minerals, and fiber. Vegetables provide a modest addition of protein, and in most cases their fat content is negligible.

One exception to the good news is carrots, which have a high GI—specifically, a 4 rating on the scale. But one carrot contains only 30 calories and 7 grams of carbohydrates, compared with about 70 calories and 13 grams of carbohydrates in a slice of bread. So carrots may be eaten in reasonable amounts, along with low GI foods. But they should *not* be eaten in large quantities alone, as in an all-carrot between-meal snack.

Winter squash (butternut and acorn) is also high on the GI scale, but summer squash is okay.

Here's a bonus: Many vegetables have so few calories per cup professional dietitians consider them "free" foods— foods which you may eat in reasonable amounts, over and above the foods planned in your regular diet. They include cabbage, celery, cucumber, green onions, lettuce, mushrooms, spinach, and zucchini. A more complete list is included in the last section of this chapter.

Here are the GI ratings for vegetables:

- *Low GI (highly desirable).* Asparagus, beans (green, wax, Italian), bean sprouts, broccoli, cabbage, cauliflower, eggplant, greens (collard, mustard, turnip), kohlrabi, leeks, mushrooms, okra, onions, pea pods, peppers (green), rutabaga, sauerkraut (but note high salt), spinach, summer squash (crookneck, zucchini), tomatoes, tomato and vegetable juices, turnips.
- *Intermediate GI (moderately desirable).* Beets.
- *High GI (less desirable).* Carrots, carrot juice, winter squash (acorn, butternut).

SHOULD YOU BOARD THE MILK WAGON?

All milk products are excellent sources of protein and calcium, but their fat content varies greatly. For purposes of weight control, dieters should focus on skim milk and low-fat milk (1 percent) products.

Dietitians divide milk products into four separate groups, based on fat content:

DIETER'S MILK CHART
(8 fl. oz. = 1 cup)

Type	Calories	Fat	Carbohydrate	Protein
Skim	90	trace	12 grams	8 grams
1 percent	100	3 grams	12 grams	8 grams
2 percent	120	5 grams	12 grams	8 grams
Whole	150	8 grams	12 grams	8 grams

The main carbohydrate in milk is a sugar called lactose Lactose has a very low Glycemic Index. Therefore, skim or low-fat milk products are excellent choices for most G-Index dieters.

Milk foods are especially useful in combination with fruit or cereal, or they can be enjoyed by themselves as a between-meal snack. Skim or low-fat milk foods include skim milk, buttermilk, and plain nonfat yogurt. Low-fat cottage cheese (nonfat, skim, or 1 percent) is an excellent low G-Index food. It is also very low in fat and is so high in protein that most nutritionists classify cottage cheese as a lean meat instead of as a milk food.

Yogurt can be a mainstay of the G-Index Diet, but there are some traps for the unwary. One of these is the high sugar content in many commercial yogurts.

An 8-ounce container of plain (unsweetened) nonfat yogurt contains 90 calories. Even adding some berries or half an apple to the yogurt only increases it by 30 calories. Artificially sweetened nonfat yogurt with fruit already added also contains only 90 to 100 calories per eight-ounce serving. Either of these approaches can give you an excellent GI class 1 combination.

But nonfat yogurt that has been made with multiple sweeteners and perhaps a bit of fruit can contain upwards of 190 calories. The increased calories are because there is actually more sweetener in these products than yogurt! Furthermore, this type of yogurt is class 4 on the GI scale because of the body's tendency to absorb the sweeteners very rapidly.

The moral is this: stick to nonfat plain yogurt, and sweeten it yourself with natural fruit, or choose a nonfat fruited yogurt with an artificial sweetener.

Frozen yogurt is an attractive snack and dessert, particularly in comparison to high-fat or high-sugar ice creams, sherbets, or sorbets. But frozen yogurts must also be selected with care. Nonfat frozen yogurts with artificial sweeteners can be useful low GI starch-equivalent snacks or desserts. But naturally sweetened frozen yogurts typically add large amounts of high GI sweeteners. This process places them in class 3 or 4, and makes them less desirable diet foods.

Frozen food products that contain Simplesse brand fat-substitute, a carbohydrate that acts as a fat, are similar. These foods may be useful for dieters *if* they have artificial or low GI sweeteners like fructose. But when the Simplesse substance is combined with high GI sweeteners, the product may trigger glucose and insulin instability. This undermines the dieter's ability to stay on a low-fat, low-calorie regimen.

Our preliminary testing of Simple Pleasures, which is a frozen dessert largely of skim milk plus the Simplesse product, with moderate amounts of sugar added, shows a reasonably good, intermediate rating on the G-Index scale.

Here are the GI ratings for low-fat milk products:

* *Low GI (highly desirable)*. Skim milk, ½ percent fat, 1 percent fat, buttermilk, evaporated skim milk, nonfat dry milk, nonfat plain yogurt, a few brands of nonfat frozen yogurt that qualify as skim-milk equivalents (the nonfat, sugar-free frozen yogurt from Honey Hills Farm, Yoglace from I Can't Believe It's Yogurt).
* *Intermediate GI (moderately desirable)*. Simple Pleasures (Simplesse-product dessert).
* *High GI (less desirable)*. None.

A note on how to cope if you can't eat dairy foods: Some people, especially after an intestinal illness, become lactose intolerant. They develop gas, cramps, and other uncomfortable symptoms when they consume milk products. This occurs because they don't produce enough lactase, an intestinal enzyme that helps digest milk sugar.

Fortunately, most people who have mild or moderate degrees of intolerance to milk and ice cream can still eat yogurt and cheese in moderate amounts without any problem. Even people who are highly intolerant of lactose milk sugar can usually take a simple pill or liquid lactase enzyme supplement just before eating a milk-containing meal. Lactase is available without prescription in most pharmacies and health food stores. Predigested, lactose-reduced milks are also available in many supermarkets.

People with these difficulties can create an excellent G-

Index Diet without any dairy products by emphasizing low GI fruits, vegetables, pastas, and legumes. Specific instructions are included in Chapter Five. In any event, dieters with this problem should consult their physician or a qualified dietitian for guidance on finding adequate milk substitutes.

HOW MEATS FIT INTO THE G-INDEX DIET

Meats, though a major source of protein, are usually also a main source of fat. And consuming fat, as you know, is the main reason for putting on extra pounds. So it's essential to select meats wisely if you want to design and maintain a low-fat diet that will be effective in taking off weight and keeping it off.

The G-Index Diet provides 25 percent or fewer calories per day from fat. This contrasts with the nearly 40 percent of calories that come from fat in the typical American diet.

The first principle to keep in mind is that the less you eat, the better. Most Americans take in considerably more protein than they need. Although this habit isn't usually harmful in itself (except for people with liver, kidney, or certain metabolic disorders), high-protein eating usually ushers in high fat consumption.

Conversely, people who want to maintain a low-fat program, and a lower calorie intake, must restrict their meat serving sizes. For example, a twelve-ounce, marbled, rib-eye steak—not an outlandish serving for a restaurant—provides roughly 1,600 calories and 70 grams of fat, or an entire day's calorie allotment on one plate—not to mention much too much fat!

Since fat contains 9 calories per gram, the 25 percent goal requires that you limit average fat intake to no more than 40 to 60 grams (360 to 540 calories) per day. Most women, short people, and less well muscled individuals should stay closer to the 40 gram level, while larger, athletic types can push the 60 gram limit. Roughly two-thirds of this fat, or 27 to 40 grams, might come from meat products while the rest comes from other fatty foods.

DAILY LIMITS FOR SPECIFIC MEAT FOODS SERVED ON THE G-INDEX DIET[1]

DAILY LIMITS FOR SPECIFIC MEAT FOODS
SERVED ON THE G-INDEX DIET

FOODS	DAILY LIMITS
EXTRA LEAN MEAT FOODS (1–5 gm fat/3 ounces)	8 ounces

Shellfish: clams, crab, lobster, scallops, shrimp
Mollusks: mussels, oysters, squid
White fish: cod, flounder, haddock, halibut, mahi mahi, monkfish, sole, red snapper, perch, pike, porgy, sea bass
Medium-fat fish: bluefish, carp, catfish, swordfish, brook trout, light chunk tuna (packed in water)
Skinless white poultry meat: chicken, turkey, Cornish hen, skinless pheasant, and quail
Egg substitute, e.g., Egg Beaters
Cottage Cheese: nonfat, low-fat, 4%
Venison
Tofu

VERY LEAN MEAT FOODS (6–8 gm fat/3 ounces)	8 ounces

Fatty fish: orange roughy, sardines, albacore tuna (packed in water)
Skinless dark poultry meat: chicken, turkey, Cornish hen
Very lean beef: flank, top round, eye round, sirloin, chipped beef, tenderloin
Very lean pork: ham steak, boiled or cured ham, loin chop
Very lean veal: loin chop, rump or sirloin roast
95% fat-free luncheon meats

---

[1]*Note:* nutritionists classify certain non-animal flesh foods as meats, e.g cottage cheese, cheese, peanut butter, and tofu (soybean curd). That is because their high protein, low carbohydrate content is similar to meats.

LEAN MEAT FOODS (9–14 gm fat/3 ounces) 5–8 ounces

High-fat fish: striped bass, canned bonito, herring, mackerel, pompano, salmon
Beef: porterhouse steak, T-bone steak, 90% lean ground
Lamb: loin chop, leg
Pork: cured butt, cured canned, smoked canned, loin chop, picnic ham (fresh or cured), tenderloin, Canadian bacon
Veal: chuck, foreshank, loin, round roast, rump roast
Skinless duck, goose
Diet cheeses (no more than 55 cal/ounce). (See page 190 for list of diet cheeses.)

MEDIUM-FAT MEAT FOODS
(15–23 gm fat/3 ounces)   5–8 ounces

Very high-fat fish: eel, lake and rainbow trout, most fried fish
Beef: cubed steak, club steak, meat loaf, rib roast, rib steak
Lamb: blade chop, rib chop, loin chop
Pork: fresh ham, picnic shoulder, sirloin, Boston butt
Veal: arm steak, blade, round cutlet, plate, rib roast, rib chop, sirloin
Organ meats: liver, heart, kidney, sweetbreads
Eggs
Cheese: part-skim (ricotta, mozzarella) reduced calorie cheeses (56–80 cal/ounce)
86% fat-free luncheon meats

HIGH-FAT MEAT FOODS
(24+ grams of fat/3 oz)
(*Do not eat except rarely and in very small amounts.*)

Beef: brisket, chuck (roast, ground, stew), corned beef, rib-eye steak, short ribs
Lamb: arm chop
Pork: blade, loin chop, sausage, shoulder, butt, spare ribs, ground pork
Veal: breast, flank, loin chop

All hot dogs (beef, pork, chicken, turkey)
Regular cheese
Regular luncheon meats (bologna, salami, pimento loaf)
Peanut butter

Your Prescription for Fat

I've referred a number of times to eating fat *prescriptively*. This means that people on the G-Index Diet may eat small quantities of fat at certain strategic times, such as for a snack or at the end of a meal, so that hunger pangs are reduced.

Fat, you'll recall, operates much as a low GI carbohydrate in that it suppresses appetite. It slows the passage of food through the stomach, thus reducing its rate of digestion and absorption. Also, adding fat to a carbohydrate reduces the rate at which the carbohydrate becomes glucose in the blood. Adding the fat reduces the effective GI of a carbohydrate food by reducing surges of blood sugar and insulin.

At the same time, however, fats must be consumed *in small amounts*. If you take in too much fat, you will put on excess pounds and increase your risk of cardiovascular disease and cancer.

All foods classified as fats are high in calories. Technically, these foods are not rated in the Glycemic Index, since they contain no carbohydrates. But because they play a critical role in the G-Index Diet, I awarded most of them a special rating of 1*. The asterisk reminds us that fats are in a separate category.

In a sense, the need for Americans to keep fat intake low is the reason I devised the G-Index Diet. You can't lose weight without getting rid of fat in your diet. At the same time, those who eat mainly high GI carbohydrates—a major staple of most weight-loss diets—find that they can't control their appetites. They are caught on the horns of a dilemma: without taking in fat, they can't stay on the diet; but with the normal, relatively high amount of fat in their diets, they can't lose weight!

The G-Index Diet represents a solution to this problem. If

you choose low GI carbohydrates, they will fulfill the blood sugar moderating function of fats, but without adding the extra calories or otherwise jeopardizing your health. Furthermore, if you eat fats in small amounts prescriptively, you'll suppress hunger even more—again, without putting on extra weight.

Other Virtues of Fat

In addition to its hunger suppression, a modest amount of fat is essential for good health. A deficiency in essential fatty acids can cause dry, scaly skin, decreased resistance to stress and disease, infertility, and fatigue.

The G-Index Diet balances fat and carbohydrate consumption so that you can enjoy good health and low weight through a low-fat eating style. The fat selections emphasize the nutritionally essential fats, which are mainly unsaturated fats that come from vegetable and seafood sources. These are the same fats that help lower cholesterol.

So how much fat should you eat each day on the G-Index Diet? The menus and recipes in Chapter Five contain the precise, small amounts you need for the set diet. If you design your own diet, follow closely the fat guidelines in the fat exchanges in Chapter Eight.

THE G-INDEX FREE FOODS

Some foods can be eaten almost without restriction on the G-Index diet because they contain minimal calories or carbohydrate. In other words, they don't increase weight, nor do they stimulate appetite. The one exception is caffeine-containing beverages—which I place in the high GI category as a less desirable food for dieters.

Here's a list of the free foods that have a low GI and are highly desirable. When there are restrictions as to amounts, those are indicated.

BEVERAGES

Bouillon (high-salt and salt-free varieties)
Broth without fat
Carbonated drinks, sugar-free
Carbonated water, club soda, or seltzer
Cocoa power, unsweetened (1 tablespoon)
Coffee or tea, decaffeinated
Drink mixes, sugar-free
Tonic water, sugar-free
Water

VEGETABLES (raw, 1 cup)

Cabbage
Celery
Chinese cabbage
Cucumber
Green onions
Hot peppers
Mushrooms
Radishes
Zucchini

SALAD GREENS

Endive
Escarole
Lettuce
Romaine
Spinach

SWEET SUBSTITUTES

Hard candy, sugar-free
Gelatin, sugar-free
Gum, sugar-free
Jam or jelly, sugar-free (2 teaspoons)

Pancake syrup, sugar-free (1–2 tablespoons)
Sugar substitutes (aspartame, saccharin)
Whipped toppings, low-calorie (2 tablespoons)

CONDIMENTS

Catsup (1 tablespoon)
Mustard
Pickles, dill, unsweetened (high-salt)
Salad dressing, very low calorie (6 calories per tablespoon)
Taco sauce (1 tablespoon)
Vinegar

A NOTE ON CAFFEINE

Caffeine is a double-edged sword. On the positive side, it stimulates the metabolism, thus promoting the burning of calories. But caffeine also stimulates the appetite, blood sugar, and insulin. In addition, there are other common negative side effects, such as overstimulation, headaches, and fatigue.

Some people develop a tolerance to the harmful effects of caffeine. Others do not. I prefer, but do not require, that those on this diet reduce or eliminate their consumption of caffeine.

This approach is especially desirable if you have noted a pattern of jitteriness, fatigue, or headaches three to four hours after eating. Also, reduce your intake if, when your usual caffeine dose is delayed, you have trouble sleeping, feel tired, become irritable, or suffer frequent headaches. In any case, people who drink the equivalent of five or more cups of coffee a day should consider a cut-back.

But if you begin to feel bad when you delay or reduce your caffeine, don't proceed further without medical supervision. Withdrawal from caffeine can be harrowing, even dangerous. There are a number of procedures or medicines that your physician may prescribe to ease the withdrawal.

Now, with this information in mind, you're prepared to make the best use of the menus, recipes, and food exchange guidelines that make up the remainder of this book.

PART II

The G-Index Diet Program

CHAPTER FIVE

The G-Index Diet

To make it easy to use the G-Index Diet, I've included in this chapter a 21-day menu plan, and in the following two chapters there are recipes, shopping lists, and other specific instructions. You'll find that almost *everything* has been done for you.

You should stay on this fixed plan for the first six weeks of the diet to build good habits and to eliminate any need to agonize over food choices. In the beginning it's important to minimize outside distractions. After you've made a good start, you'll be ready to move on to Part II, designing your *own* G-Index Diet.

As you use the 21-day program, there are some fundamental rules you should know.

Rule 1. Don't skip meals or snacks. Every day, try to eat all three meals and a mid-afternoon and evening snack. Do not eat less than the planned amounts or you may feel hungry later. People who eat a good G-Index breakfast usually do not require a mid-morning snack. But if you wish, you may add a mid-morning snack from the G-Index snack list in Chapter Seven.

Rule 2. Be especially conscientious about sticking to the G-Index Diet at snack time. Avoid substituting snacks with a high GI. Remember, foods with a high GI will increase hunger and encourage poor food choices at the next meal.

Rule 3. If you slip and eat a high G-Index food between meals, combine it with about 50 calories of fat. This advice may seem to be making a bad situation worse. But this prescriptive use of fat will help stave off the hunger that will be caused by a high GI food. For example, you might include one-half tablespoon of natural peanut butter or one-half ounce of cheese. The fat may add a few extra calories, but at least you will avoid triggering the vicious cycle of rising blood sugar, insulin, and appetite.

Rule 4. You are allowed to use one or two teaspoons of sugar daily as a sweetener, or up to four teaspoons of fructose. I don't encourage sugar use, but modest amounts of sucrose and fructose are less disruptive for your diet than one slice of commercial bread.

Caution: Eating sweets regularly, especially in large amounts, will dull your perception of sweetness and cause you to want more sweets to obtain the same level of satisfaction. In contrast, after you've been on the G-Index for only about three weeks, you'll find that your perceptions of sweetness will be sharpened and the sugars in fresh fruits and vegetables will be more satisfying.

Rule 5. Limit your fats, including the ones you use prescriptively. Refer to the previous chapter for guidelines. Remember, this is a low-fat diet, with 25 percent of daily calories coming from fats. You don't want to subvert it by failing to pay close enough attention to the fats you use to ward off appetite.

Rule 6. Cut back on caffeine. Caffeine is a double-edged sword. It promotes weight loss by stimulating the body's metabolism. But it also hinders hunger control by undermining the stability of blood sugar, insulin, and appetite. Most people do better on a diet by minimizing its use or eliminating it entirely.

Rule 7. Drink a minimum of eight 8-ounce glasses of water, plus other fluids, every day. Add one extra glass per day for every 25 pounds you need to lose.

Rule 8. Don't punish yourself if you violate the diet. If you eat prohibited foods or go on a binge, don't feel guilty or try to compensate by skipping meals or snacks. With this sort of response, you'll likely fall into even worse eating habits. Instead, you can undo much of the damage by devoting twenty-four hours to a regimen of all low GI, low-fat foods. This will make you feel better psychologically and will also help restore the G-Index Diet metabolic balance.

Rule 9. Expect some minor "withdrawal" discomfort during the first three days you go off high G-Index foods. You must give the diet a full three weeks to "settle in." Mild intestinal gas may increase temporarily owing to the relatively high fiber content of the G-Index approach.

Or if you have a latent lactase-enzyme deficiency (an intolerance of lactose, or milk sugar), you may experience gas when you consume milk products. People with this problem will probably have to cut back, at least to some extent, on dairy products. It will be helpful to consult a qualified dietitian for advice about foods that are good substitutes for milk, yogurt, and similar products. Among other things, you may need a calcium supplement. For specific instructions, see page 67 on the milk family of foods.

Rule 10. Regular, moderate endurance exercise will increase your weight loss and help you stay on the diet.

Exercise isn't required for you to lose weight on this diet. But as I've already indicated, it can be an important component in both weight loss and maintenance of a lower weight. Both aerobic or endurance exercises (such as walking and jogging) and muscle-building programs can help. The greater your muscle mass, the greater your body's ability to burn fat by stimulating your metabolic rate.

Rule 11. Most people on the G-Index Diet don't need vitamin or mineral supplements. One exception is that people who are milk intolerant will need a calcium supplement (see Rule 22). Otherwise, there are sufficient nutrients in these menus and recipes to fulfill all standard nutritional allowances.

Rule 12. Select the calorie level that's best for you.

Nearly all women and small men should use the 1,200 calorie diet for weight loss; most other men should use the 1,500 calorie plan. For weight maintenance nearly all women and small men should use the 1,500 calorie diet while most other men should use the 1,800 calorie diet.

Larger men who want to maintain a weight of 180 pounds or more—or very athletic men or women—may find that they need to add calories to the 1,800-calorie diet to keep from losing too many pounds. The extra foods may be taken from the exchange list in Chapter Eight and consumed as either additional snacks or part of a larger meal.

In general, both your weight-loss and your weight-maintenance strategy must be tailored to your particular needs. Watch the rate at which you are losing. If you're taking off about 2 to 3 pounds a week, you're on the right track. Also, if you're maintaining your ideal weight at a particular calorie level, stick to it!

Rule 13. Assemble the basic equipment you need to make the recipes. Other than the usual utensils and other paraphernalia available in most kitchens, little in the way of extra equipment is required. But you might want to have these items if they aren't already part of your cooking materials:

- A nonstick frying pan or skillet
- A nonstick cooking spray
- A microwave oven

Rule 14. Utilize the Shortcuts, Lightning Alternatives, and other optional suggestions in the recipes if you're in a hurry or lack certain equipment. The recipes contain a number of quick preparation suggestions, such as using commercial frozen foods to substitute for various ingredients. Feel free to use these when necessary because they have appropriate nutrients and fit in well with the G-Index approach.

Rule 15. Choose sugar-free items from your supermarket whenever possible. A number of the foods in these menus and recipes—such as gelatin, applesauce, and puddings—enhance the impact of the G-Index Diet if they are the sugar-free variety. Always check for this option in your supermarket.

Rule 16. Nonfat yogurt should always be either plain or fruited with an artificial sweetener. Here's a rule of thumb: You probably have the right product if an 8-ounce serving contains only 90 to 100 calories. If there are more calories, sugar is probably present and that means excessive glucose and a high GI.

Rule 17. Low-calorie salad dressings should contain no more than 10 calories per tablespoon.

Rule 18. Whole-grain bread or other whole wheat products should be low on the Glycemic Index. You can find more extensive guidelines in Chapter Four and Chapter Eight, but remember that breads and bread products should be predominantly whole grain, primarily sprouted or cracked grain, 100 percent coarsely stone-ground whole wheat, rye, or pumpernickel. It's acceptable to use fine-textured 100 percent stone-ground whole wheat bread, but the other types are preferable. Pita bread is an excellent choice; 100 percent stoneground is preferred.

Rule 19. Diet cheese should be no more than 55 calories per ounce and should be at least 95 percent fat-free. Many cheeses that are labelled as reduced calorie, low-fat, light, etc., have more than 55 calories per ounce. Check the labels.

Rule 20. Eggs should be cooked with nonstick cooking spray.

Rule 21. You may substitute equal amounts of whole fruit for fruit juice, or fruit juice for whole fruit. Whole fruit is preferred because the fiber in it fills you up more, and also you will eat it more slowly because you have to ''work'' as you chew it. But the Glycemic Index for juice and whole fruit is equivalent. So long as you choose comparable amounts (see appropriate items under the fruit exchanges in Chapter Eight), you can exchange the two forms of fruit as desired.

Rule 22. People who are lactose (milk sugar) intolerant must make certain adjustments in the diet. First, it's essential to seek guidance from a physician or qualified dietitian. Then one of the following may be substituted for each 8-ounce glass of milk or serving of yogurt (usually with a 300 mg. calcium supplement, as directed by your physician):

- 8 ounces of lactose-free nonfat milk (no calcium supplement necessary)
- 8 ounces of skim milk or nonfat yogurt with lactase drops or tablets (no calcium supplement)
- 2 ounces of diet cheese

- ½ cup of nonfat cottage cheese
- ½ cup egg substitute, plus ¼ cup of low G-Index fruit juice
- ½ cup of a low GI cereal, such as Fiber One, plus ¼ cup of fruit juice
- 1 slice of whole-grain bread with fruit butter or sugar-free jelly
- 2 ounces of roasted skinless chicken breast.

Rule 23. Reduced-calorie mayonnaise should contain no more than 20 calories per tablespoon.

HOW MUCH WEIGHT CAN YOU EXPECT TO LOSE?

The following fixed menus and recipes have been designed to allow the average woman to lose 2 to 3 pounds per week, and the average man 3 to 4 pounds per week, at the 1,200-calorie level. This means that a typical woman could lose 18 pounds if she stays on the fixed menus for the recommended six weeks, and the typical man could lose 24 pounds.

In general, however, how much weight a given person can lose depends on his or her physical size, development of muscle tissue, and activity level. A very small, physically inactive woman might lose less than 2 to 3 pounds per week, while a 200-pound athletic man with well-developed muscles might lose considerably more than 3 to 4 pounds per week.

After the first six weeks, further weight loss can be achieved by either continuing the fixed program or designing your own diet, as described in Part III of this book. Or if you make your desired weight in the first six weeks, you can *maintain* it *permanently*—without hunger—by increasing your food intake with a 1,500-calorie G-Index Diet if you're a woman or a 1,800-calorie G-Index Diet if you're a man.

Introduction to the Menus

To keep the menu instructions brief and readable we have used certain food terms as a kind of shorthand for what really should be more complicated instructions. For the purpose of this menu please keep the following additional instructions in mind.

When we describe a dessert or snack food as *"low calorie,"* e.g., low calorie pudding, we mean the sugar-free version.

When we say 100 percent *whole grain* we mean for the purpose of this menu several types of low G-Index, less-refined breads most of which, strictly speaking, are not really 100 percent whole grain. Acceptable breads include those made from predominantly whole grain, sprouted or cracked grain, 100 percent coarsely ground whole wheat, coarse whole grain rye, pumpernickel rye, or pita bread. Fine texture 100 percent stone-ground whole wheat bread is acceptable, but less preferred.

By *yogurt* we mean plain or fruited yogurt with artificial sweetener. 8 ounces equals 90–100 calories. Frozen yogurt also means the non-fat, non-sugar variety.

Low calorie salad dressing means salad dressing with no more than 10 calories per tablespoon.

By *diet cheese* we mean cheeses that contain no more than 55 calories per ounce. These are 95 percent fat-free.

Substitutions: If you are lactose intolerant or unable to take a milk or yogurt serving, you may substitute for each 8 ounce milk or yogurt serving any of the dairy or non-dairy options listed in Rule 22 on page 83.

If you do not like a particular meal, you may substitute the same meal from another day. Don't do this too often. We balanced the nutrients for each full day. One dinner is not nutritionally identical to another. However, as a practical matter you're much better off substituting than you would be by either skipping a meal or going off your diet. Since each day's menu is nutritionally complete you *may* repeat the *complete* meal plan of favorite days as often as you wish.

You may also make various common sense substitutions. For example, on day one if you would not eat clam sauce with your linguini, a roughly comparable, no sugar added substitute could be Season's marinara sauce (kosher), or Hunt's Home Style Traditional spaghetti sauce. When fruit

or fruit juice are offered, you may substitute any other fruit
or fruit juice in the equivalent amount listed on the fruit
exchange list, page 293. However, the fruit or fruit juice
substituted must have the same or lower G-Index rating as
the fruit or fruit juice you are omitting. Similarly you may
also substitute among vegetables.

Note: We occasionally use brand names when these fit
our nutritional requirements. Usually, but not always, other
brands of similar products are also okay. Equivalent, acceptable brands are listed on the Exchange Lists, page 275.

Menu entries written in all capital letters are those with
recipes listed in Chapter Six, page 128.

Measures: There is a complete list of measures and their
equivalents on pages 193–195. However, it might be convenient to list a few key measures here:

1 fluid ounce = ⅛ cup = 2 tablespoons = 6 teaspoons
1 cup = 8 ounces
1 tablespoon = 3 teaspoons = ½ ounce

THE 21 DAYS OF MENUS

DAY 1

Meal	Food Item	1,200 Cal	1,500 Cal	1,800 Cal
Breakfast	whole-grain bread	1 slice	1 slice	1 slice
	peanut butter or cheese (Swiss, American, Monterey Jack, cheddar)	1 tbs	1 tbs	1 tbs
		1 oz	1 oz	1 oz
	orange juice	4 oz	4 oz	8 oz
	or blueberries	¾ cup	¾ cup	1½ cups

Meal	Food Item	1,200 Cal	1,500 Cal	1,800 Cal
	skim milk or nonfat yogurt	4 oz	8 oz	8 oz
	decaf coffee or tea	as desired	as desired	as desired
	skim milk or light nondairy creamer	2 oz 1 oz	2 oz 1 oz	2 oz 1 oz
Lunch	Ry Krisp crackers	4	4	4
	SPICY CHEESE DIP[1]	½ cup	½ cup	¾ cup
	bell pepper strips	1 cup	1 cup	1 cup
	cantaloupe or citrus sections	1 cup ¾ cup	1 cup ¾ cup	1 cup ¾ cup
	skim milk or nonfat yogurt	—	—	4 oz
	water or decaf diet beverage	as desired	as desired	as desired
Snack	Ry Krisp crackers with fruit butter or sugar-free jelly (optional)	4 3 tsp	4 3 tsp	8 4 tsp
	water or decaf diet beverage	as desired	as desired	as desired
Dinner	linguine	1 cup	1½ cups	1½ cups
	White clam sauce, no sugar added (e.g., Progresso)	½ cup	¾ cup	¾ cup

[1]*Note:* Recipes in capital letters appear in Chapter Six, page 128.

Meal	Food Item	1,200 Cal	1,500 Cal	1,800 Cal
	MARINATED LONDON BROIL	2 oz	3 oz	3 oz
	steamed broccoli or asparagus	½ cup	1 cup	1½ cups
	with lemon & garlic	as desired	as desired	as desired
	with olive oil	1 tsp	1 tsp	2 tsp
	endive & romaine salad	3 cups	3 cups	3 cups
	with low-calorie dressing	2 tbs	2 tbs	2 tbs
	cantaloupe	1 cup	1 cup	1 cup
	or baked apple with cinnamon	1 small	1 small	1 small
	water or decaf diet beverage	as desired	as desired	as desired
Snack	FRUIT FRAPPE	½ cup	1 cup	1 cup

DAY 2

Meal	Food Item	1,200 Cal	1,500 Cal	1,800 Cal
Breakfast	Extra Fiber All-Bran or Fiber One cereal	1 cup	1 cup	1⅓ cups
	cantaloupe	1 cup	2 cups	2 cups
	or pear	1 small	1 large	1 large
	skim milk or nonfat yogurt	8 oz	8 oz	8 oz
	decaf coffee or tea	as desired	as desired	as desired

Meal	Food Item	1,200 Cal	1,500 Cal	1,800 Cal
	skim milk or light nondairy	2 oz	2 oz	2 oz
	creamer	1 oz	1 oz	1 oz
Lunch	whole-grain bread	1 slice	2 slices	2 slices
	leftover LONDON BROIL	2 oz	3 oz	3 oz
	lettuce	as desired	as desired	as desired
	mayonnaise (light), (optional)	1 tbs	1 tbs	1 tbs
	tomato, cucumber, & oregano salad with low-calorie	2 cups	3 cups	3 cups
	dressing	2 tbs	2 tbs	2 tbs
	apple or orange	1 small	1 small	1 small
	water or decaf diet beverage	as desired	as desired	as desired
Snack	graham cracker squares	3	3	3
	with (light or whipped) cream cheese	½ oz	½ oz	½ oz
	with fruit butter or sugar-free jelly (optional)	4 tsp	4 tsp	4 tsp
	apple or pear	—	1 small	1 small
	skim milk or nonfat yogurt	—	—	4 oz
	water or decaf diet beverage	as desired	as desired	as desired

Meal	Food Item	1,200 Cal	1,500 Cal	1,800 Cal
Dinner	PEA SOUP (e.g., Health Valley, Pritikin, or Progresso	1 cup	1 cup	1 cup
	SAUTÉED SCALLOPS MEDITER-RANEAN	4 oz	4 oz	6 oz
	BRAISED LEEKS	2 leeks	2 leeks	4 leeks
	tossed green salad with low-calorie dressing	3 cups	3 cups	3 cups
		2 tbs	2 tbs	2 tbs
	fresh fruit cup or blueberries	¾ cup	¾ cup	1½ cups
	water or decaf diet beverage	as desired	as desired	as desired
Snack	low-calorie pudding	½ cup	½ cup	½ cup
	light whipped topping (optional)	2 tbs	2 tbs	2 tbs
	water or decaf diet beverage	as desired	as desired	as desired

DAY 3

Meal	Food Item	1,200 Cal	1,500 Cal	1,800 Cal
Breakfast	whole-grain bread	1 slice	1 slice	1 slice

Meal	Food Item	1,200 Cal	1,500 Cal	1,800 Cal
	egg, poached, boiled, or scrambled	1 large	1 large	1 large
	banana	½	1	1
	or grapefruit juice	4 oz	8 oz	8 oz
	skim milk or nonfat yogurt	8 oz	8 oz	8 oz
	decaf coffee or tea	as desired	as desired	as desired
	skim milk	2 oz	2 oz	2 oz
	or light nondairy creamer	1 oz	1 oz	1 oz
Lunch	whole wheat pita pocket	1 oz (1 small)	1 oz (1 small)	2 oz (1 large)
	with HUMMUS-TAHINI SPREAD	¼ cup	¼ cup	½ cup
	with alfalfa sprouts	½ cup	½ cup	1 cup
	cantaloupe	2 cups	2 cups	2 cups
	or banana	1	1	1
	water or decaf diet beverage	as desired	as desired	as desired
Snack	Ry Krisp crackers	4	4	4
	with (light or whipped) cream cheese	½ oz	½ oz	½ oz
	with fruit butter or sugar-free jelly (optional)	4 tsp	4 tsp	4 tsp
	water or decaf diet beverage	as desired	as desired	as desired

Meal	Food Item	1,200 Cal	1,500 Cal	1,800 Cal
Dinner	potato, boiled, with skin	1 small	1 small	1 small
	BREAST OF CHICKEN ROSEMARY	3 oz	4 oz	4 oz
	sautéed spinach with garlic	1½ cups	2 cups	2 cups
	with olive oil	1 tsp	2 tsp	2 tsp
	tossed green salad	3 cups	3 cups	3 cups
	with low-calorie dressing	2 tbs	2 tbs	2 tbs
	apple or pear	1 small	1 small	1 small
	water or decaf diet beverage	as desired	as desired	as desired
Snack	graham cracker squares	—	3	3
	AMBROSIA	½ cup	½ cup	1 cup
	or applesauce	½ cup	½ cup	1 cup
	skim milk or nonfat yogurt	4 oz	8 oz	8 oz

DAY 4

Meal	Food Item	1,200 Cal	1,500 Cal	1,800 Cal
Breakfast	Extra Fiber All-Bran or Fiber One Cereal	⅔ cup	1⅓ cup	1⅓ cup
	blueberries	¾ cup	¾ cup	¾ cup
	or apple	1 small	1 small	1 small
	skim milk or nonfat yogurt	8 oz	8 oz	8 oz

Meal	Food Item	1,200 Cal	1,500 Cal	1,800 Cal
	decaf coffee or tea	as desired	as desired	as desired
	skim milk	2 oz	2 oz	2 oz
	or light nondairy creamer	1 oz	1 oz	1 oz
Lunch	Ry Krisp crackers	2	2	4
	TASTY CRABMEAT SALAD	½ cup	½ cup	½ cup
	with iceberg lettuce	as desired	as desired	as desired
	bell pepper strips	1 cup	1 cup	2 cups
	or celery stalks	3	3	3
	peach or pear	1 small	1 small	1 large
	water or decaf diet beverage	as desired	as desired	as desired
Snack	dry-roasted almonds	6 whole	6 whole	6 whole
	nonfat yogurt	4 oz	4 oz	8 oz
	water or decaf diet beverage	as desired	as desired	as desired
Dinner	LIGHT MACARONI AND CHEESE	1½ cups	1½ cups	1½ cups
	stewed tomatoes, basil, & oregano	½ cup	1 cup	1 cup
	tossed green salad	3 cups	3 cups	3 cups
	with low-calorie dressing	2 tbs	2 tbs	2 tbs

Meal	Food Item	1,200 Cal	1,500 Cal	1,800 Cal
	orange or baked apple with cinnamon	1 small	1 large	1 large
	water or decaf diet beverage	as desired	as desired	as desired
Snack	cheese (Swiss, American, Monterey Jack, cheddar)	1 oz	2 oz	3 oz
	peach or apple	1 small	1 small	1 small
	skim milk or nonfat yogurt	—	4 oz	8 oz

DAY 5

Meal	Food Item	1,200 Cal	1,500 Cal	1,800 Cal
Breakfast	whole-grain bread	1 slice	1 slice	1 slice
	low-sodium ham or diet cheese	1 oz	1 oz	1 oz
	peach or orange	1 small	1 small	1 small
	skim milk or nonfat yogurt	4 oz	8 oz	8 oz
	decaf coffee or tea	as desired	as desired	as desired
	skim milk	2 oz	2 oz	2 oz
	or light nondairy creamer	1 oz	1 oz	1 oz
Lunch	whole-grain bread	2 slices	2 slices	2 slices

Meal	Food Item	1,200 Cal	1,500 Cal	1,800 Cal
	roasted turkey breast	2 oz	2 oz	2 oz
	with tomato	1 slice	1 slice	1 slice
	with lettuce	as desired	as desired	as desired
	with reduced-calorie mayonnaise	1 tbs	1 tbs	1 tbs
	tomato, cucumber, & oregano salad	2 cups	2 cups	4 cups
	with low-calorie dressing	2 tbs	2 tbs	2 tbs
	apple	1 small	1 small	1 small
	or banana	½	½	½
	water or decaf diet beverage	as desired	as desired	as desired
Snack	dry-roasted almonds	—	6 whole	6 whole
	skim milk or nonfat yogurt	8 oz	8 oz	8 oz
	water or decaf diet beverage	as desired	as desired	as desired
Dinner	COUNTRY-STYLE MINESTRONE	1 cup	1 cup	1 cup
	CHICKEN CUTLET LILLIAN	2½ oz	2½ oz	5 oz
	GRILLED EGGPLANT (See GRILLED VEGETABLES)	½ cup	1 cup	1 cup
	spinach salad	3 cups	3 cups	3 cups
	with low-calorie dressing	2 tbs	2 tbs	2 tbs

Meal	Food Item	1,200 Cal	1,500 Cal	1,800 Cal
	peach or apple water or decaf	1 small	1 small	1 small
	diet beverage	as desired	as desired	as desired
Snack	graham cracker squares	3	6	6
	with fruit butter or sugar-free jelly (optional)	1 tbs	1 tbs	1 tbs
	pear	1 small	1 small	1 large
	or banana	½	½	1
	skim milk or nonfat yogurt	—	4 oz	4 oz

DAY 6

Meal	Food Item	1,200 Cal	1,500 Cal	1,800 Cal
Breakfast	old-fashioned cooked oatmeal	½ cup	½ cup	½ cup
	grapefruit	½	1	1
	or applesauce	½ cup	1 cup	1 cup
	FRUIT FRAPPE	½ cup	½ cup	½ cup
	decaf coffee or tea	as desired	as desired	as desired
	skim milk	2 oz	2 oz	2 oz
	or light nondairy creamer	1 oz	1 oz	1 oz
Lunch	low-sodium chicken broth (Health Valley, Campbell's)	—	1 cup	1 cup

Meal	Food Item	1,200 Cal	1,500 Cal	1,800 Cal
	whole-grain bread	1 slice	1 slice	1 slice
	leftover CHICKEN CUTLET	2½ oz	2½ oz	2½ oz
	with tomato	1 slice	1 slice	1 slice
	with lettuce	as desired	as desired	as desired
	pear or orange	1 large	1 large	1 large
	water or decaf diet beverage	as desired	as desired	as desired
Snack	Ry Krisp crackers	4	4	4
	with fruit butter or sugar-free jelly (optional)	4 tsp	4 tsp	4 tsp
	water or decaf diet beverage	as desired	as desired	as desired
Dinner	spaghetti	1 cup	1 cup	1½ cups
	MEATBALLS PARMIGIANA	1	1	2
	tomato sauce	¼ cup	¼ cup	½ cup
	sautéed string beans, parsley, & thyme	½ cup	1 cup	1½ cups
	with olive oil	2 tsp	1 tbs	1 tbs
	endive & romaine salad	3 cups	3 cups	3 cups
	with low-calorie dressing	2 tbs	2 tbs	2 tbs
	fresh fruit cup	¾ cup	¾ cup	1½ cups
	water or decaf diet beverage	as desired	as desired	as desired
Snack	gelatin	1 cup	1 cup	1 cup

Meal	Food Item	1,200 Cal	1,500 Cal	1,800 Cal
	light whipped topping (optional)	2 tbs	2 tbs	2 tbs
	skim milk	4 oz	8 oz	8 oz

DAY 7

Meal	Food Item	1,200 Cal	1,500 Cal	1,800 Cal
Breakfast	whole-grain bread	1 slice	1 slice	1 slice
	SCRAMBLED EGG WITH SALSA	1 large egg	1 large egg	1 large egg
	orange juice	4 oz	4 oz	4 oz
	or orange	1 small	1 small	1 small
	diet margarine	—	—	2 tbs
	skim milk or nonfat yogurt	4 oz	8 oz	8 oz
	decaf coffee or tea	as desired	as desired	as desired
	skim milk	2 oz	2 oz	2 oz
	or light nondairy creamer	1 oz	1 oz	1 oz
Lunch	Ry Krisp crackers	4	4	4
	CHEF'S SALAD with low-calorie dressing	2 cups 2 tbs	2 cups 2 tbs	3 cups 2 tbs
	pear	1 small	1 small	1 large
	or banana	½	½	1
	water or decaf diet beverage	as desired	as desired	as desired

Snack	low-calorie pudding (Dezerta, sugar-free Jell-O)	½ cup	½ cup	½ cup
	or nonfat yogurt	8 oz	8 oz	8 oz
	water or decaf diet beverage	as desired	as desired	as desired
Dinner	FILLET OF COD MILKY WAY	4 oz	4 oz	6 oz
	steamed couscous or rice	½ cup	1 cup	1 cup
	RATATOUILLE	½ cup	1 cup	1 cup
	tossed green salad	3 cups	3 cups	3 cups
	with low-calorie dressing	2 tbs	2 tbs	2 tbs
	fresh berries	¾ cup	¾ cup	¾ cup
	or baked apple with cinnamon	1 small	1 small	1 small
	with light whipped topping (optional)	2 tbs	2 tbs	2 tbs
	water or decaf diet beverage	as desired	as desired	as desired
Snack	graham cracker squares	3	3	3
	with fruit butter or sugar-free jelly (optional)	1 tbs	1 tbs	1 tbs
	grapefruit juice	4 oz	8 oz	8 oz

DAY 8

Meal	Food Item	1,200 Cal	1,500 Cal	1,800 Cal
Breakfast	whole-grain bread	1 slice	2 slices	2 slices
	peanut butter	2 tbs	3 tbs	3 tbs
	or cheese (Swiss, American, Monterey Jack, cheddar)	2 oz	3 oz	3 oz
	orange juice	4 oz	4 oz	4 oz
	or orange	1 small	1 small	1 small
	skim milk or nonfat yogurt	4 oz	4 oz	4 oz
	decaf coffee or tea	as desired	as desired	as desired
	skim milk	2 oz	2 oz	2 oz
	or light nondairy creamer	1 oz	1 oz	1 oz
Lunch	whole wheat pita pocket	1 small (1 oz)	1 small (1 oz)	1 small (1 oz)
	with tasty tuna salad (see TASTY CRABMEAT SALAD recipe Day 4)	½ cup	½ cup	½ cup
	with bean sprouts	1 cup	1 cup	1 cup
	strawberries	1¼ cups	1¼ cups	1¼ cups
	or tangerines	2	2	2
	water or decaf diet beverage	as desired	as desired	as desired
Snack	graham cracker squares	3	3	3
	with light or whipped cream cheese	—	½ oz	½ oz

Meal	Food Item	1,200 Cal	1,500 Cal	1,800 Cal
	with fruit butter or sugar-free jelly (optional)	1 tbs	1 tbs	1 tbs
	skim milk or nonfat yogurt	—	4 oz	8 oz
	water or decaf diet beverage	as desired	as desired	as desired
Dinner	GREEN LASAGNA	1½ cups	1½ cups	2½ cups
	leftover ratatouille	1 cup	1 cup	1½ cups
	tossed green salad	3 cups	3 cups	3 cups
	with low-calorie dressing	2 tbs	2 tbs	2 tbs
	fresh fruit cup	¾ cup	1½ cups	1½ cups
	water or decaf diet beverage	as desired	as desired	as desired
Snack	FRUIT FRAPPE	1 cup	1 cup	1 cup

DAY 9

Meal	Food Item	1,200 Cal	1,500 Cal	1,800 Cal
Breakfast	Extra Fiber All-Bran or Fiber One cereal	⅔ cup	⅔ cup	1⅓ cup
	strawberries	1¼ cups	1¼ cups	1¼ cups
	or banana	½	½	½
	skim milk or nonfat yogurt	4 oz	4 oz	4 oz
	decaf coffee or tea	as desired	as desired	as desired

Meal	Food Item	1,200 Cal	1,500 Cal	1,800 Cal
	skim milk or light nondairy creamer	2 oz 1 oz	2 oz 1 oz	2 oz 1 oz
Lunch	whole-grain bread	1 slice	2 slices	2 slices
	DEVILED EGGS WITH TOFU	4 halves	4 halves	4 halves
	lettuce, tomato, & cucumber salad	3 cups	3 cups	3 cups
	with low-calorie dressing	2 tbs	2 tbs	2 tbs
	nectarine or apple	1 small	1 small	1 small
	water or decaf diet beverage	as desired	as desired	as desired
Snack	unsalted peanuts	20 small	20 small	40 small
	skim milk or nonfat yogurt	8 oz	8 oz	8 oz
Dinner	sweet potato	⅔ cup	⅔ cup	⅔ cup
	broiled flank steak	3 oz	4 oz	5 oz
	STEAMED BROCCOLI or ASPARAGUS (See STEAMED VEGETABLES)	1 cup	1½ cups	2 cups
	with lemon & garlic	as desired	as desired	as desired
	with diet margarine	1 tbs	2 tbs	2 tbs
	nectarine	1 small	1 large	1 large
	or banana	½	1	1

Meal	Food Item	1,200 Cal	1,500 Cal	1,800 Cal
	water or decaf diet beverage	as desired	as desired	as desired
Snack	graham cracker squares	3	3	3
	with light or whipped cream cheese	½ oz	½ oz	½ oz
	with fruit butter or sugar-free jelly (optional)	1 tbs	1 tbs	1 tbs
	apple or baked apple with cinnamon	1 small	1 small	1 large
	skim milk or nonfat yogurt	—	4 oz	8 oz

DAY 10

Meal	Food Item	1,200 Cal	1,500 Cal	1,800 Cal
Breakfast	whole-grain bread	1 slice	1 slice	1 slice
	low-sodium ham	1 oz	1 oz	2 oz
	or diet cheese	1 oz	1 oz	2 oz
	pear	1 small	1 small	1 small
	or banana	½	½	½
	skim milk or nonfat yogurt	4 oz	8 oz	8 oz
	decaf coffee or tea	as desired	as desired	as desired
	skim milk or light nondairy creamer	2 oz	2 oz	2 oz
		1 oz	1 oz	1 oz

Meal	Food Item	1,200 Cal	1,500 Cal	1,800 Cal
Lunch	whole-grain bread	1 slice	2 slices	2 slices
	roasted turkey breast	1 oz	2 oz	2 oz
	with lettuce	as desired	as desired	as desired
	with tomato	1 slice	1 slice	1 slice
	with mayonnaise (light)	1 tbs	1 tbs	1 tbs
	cucumber & dill salad	2 cups	2 cups	2 cups
	with low-calorie dressing	2 tbs	2 tbs	2 tbs
	nectarine or apple	1 small	1 small	1 small
	water or decaf diet beverage	as desired	as desired	as desired
Snack	unsalted peanuts	20 small	20 small	20 small
	skim milk or nonfat yogurt	8 oz	8 oz	8 oz
	water or decaf diet beverage	as desired	as desired	as desired
Dinner	SESAME CHICKEN KABOBS	3 oz	3 oz	3 oz
	couscous or rice	⅔ cup	⅔ cup	1 cup
	WILTED BOK CHOY	1 cup	2 cups	2 cups
	with olive oil	1 tsp	2 tsp	1 tbs
	tossed green salad	3 cups	3 cups	3 cups
	with low-calorie dressing	2 tbs	2 tbs	2 tbs
	fresh fruit cup	¾ cup	1½ cups	1½ cups
	water or decaf diet beverage	as desired	as desired	as desired

Meal	Food Item	1,200 Cal	1,500 Cal	1,800 Cal
Snack	graham cracker squares with fruit butter or sugar-free	3	3	3
	jelly (optional)	1 tbs	1 tbs	1 tbs
	apple juice	4 oz	4 oz	8 oz
	or applesauce	½ cup	½ cup	1 cup
	skim milk or nonfat yogurt	—	—	4 oz

DAY 11

Meal	Food Item	1,200 Cal	1,500 Cal	1,800 Cal
Breakfast	Extra Fiber All-Bran or Fiber One	⅔ cup	⅔ cup	1⅓ cups
	apple	1 small	1 small	1 large
	or banana	½	½	1
	skim milk or nonfat yogurt	8 oz	8 oz	8 oz
	decaf coffee or tea	as desired	as desired	as desired
	skim milk or light nondairy	2 oz	2 oz	2 oz
	creamer	1 oz	1 oz	1 oz
Lunch	whole-wheat pita pocket with tasty chicken salad (see TASTY CRABMEAT SALAD	1 small (1 oz)	1 large (2 oz)	1 large (2 oz)
	recipe)	½ cup	¾ cup	1 cup

Meal	Food Item	1,200 Cal	1,500 Cal	1,800 Cal
	with diced tomato	¼ cup	¼ cup	¼ cup
	cantaloupe	1 cup	1 cup	1 cup
	or pear	1 small	1 small	1 small
	water or decaf diet beverage	as desired	as desired	as desired
Snack	graham cracker squares	3	3	4
	with light or whipped cream cheese	½ oz	½ oz	1 oz
	with fruit butter or sugar-free jelly (optional)	3 tsp	3 tsp	4 tsp
	skim milk or nonfat yogurt	—	—	4 oz
	water or decaf diet beverage	as desired	as desired	as desired
Dinner	PASTA PRIMAVERA	2 cups	2 cups	2 cups
	90% lean hamburger patty	3 oz	4 oz	4 oz
	with catsup	1 tbs	1 tbs	1 tbs
	tossed green salad	3 cups	3 cups	3 cups
	with tomato	1 large	1 large	1 large
	with olives	5 large	5 large	5 large
	with low-calorie dressing	2 tbs	2 tbs	2 tbs
	fresh fruit cup	¾ cup	¾ cup	¾ cup
	water or decaf diet beverage	as desired	as desired	as desired
Snack	mixed berries or fresh fruit cup	¾ cup	1½ cups	1½ cups

Meal	Food Item	1,200 Cal	1,500 Cal	1,800 Cal
	light whipped topping (optional)	2 tbs	2 tbs	2 tbs
	skim milk or nonfat yogurt	4 oz	8 oz	8 oz
	water or decaf diet beverage	as desired	as desired	as desired

DAY 12

Meal	Food Item	1,200 Cal	1,500 Cal	1,800 Cal
Breakfast	whole-grain bread	1 slice	1 slice	1 slice
	low-sodium boiled ham	1 oz	1 oz	2 oz
	or diet cheese	1 oz	1 oz	2 oz
	orange juice	4 oz	4 oz	4 oz
	or orange	1 small	1 small	1 small
	skim milk or nonfat yogurt	4 oz	8 oz	8 oz
	decaf coffee or tea	as desired	as desired	as desired
	skim milk	2 oz	2 oz	2 oz
	or light nondairy creamer	1 oz	1 oz	1 oz
Lunch	pizza melt (see BACON & CHEESE MELT recipe) with whole-grain bread	1 slice	1 slice	1 slice
	with part-skim mozzarella cheese	1 oz	2 oz	3 oz

Meal	Food Item	1,200 Cal	1,500 Cal	1,800 Cal
	with tomato	1 slice	1 slice	1 slice
	with dried oregano	as desired	as desired	as desired
	tomato & cucumber salad	2 cups	3 cups	3 cups
	with low-calorie dressing	2 tbs	2 tbs	2 tbs
	pear or apple	1 small	1 small	1 large
	water or decaf diet beverage	as desired	as desired	as desired
Snack	skim milk or nonfat yogurt	4 oz	4 oz	8 oz
	pear or apple	1 small	1 large	1 large
	water or decaf diet beverage	as desired	as desired	as desired
Dinner	CHICKEN WITH MARKET VEGETABLES	1½ cups	2¼ cups	2¼ cups
	CURRIED COUSCOUS	⅔ cup	1 cup	1⅓ cups
	with margarine (diet)	1 tbs	1½ tbs	2½ tbs
	tossed green salad	3 cups	3 cups	3 cups
	with low-calorie dressing	2 tbs	2 tbs	2 tbs
	nectarine or orange	1 small	1 small	1 small
	water or decaf diet beverage	as desired	as desired	as desired
Snack	APPLES 'N' OATS MUFFIN	1	1	1

Meal	Food Item	1,200 Cal	1,500 Cal	1,800 Cal
	with fruit butter or sugar-free jelly (optional)	1 tbs	1 tbs	1 tbs
	water or decaf diet beverage	as desired	as desired	as desired

DAY 13

Meal	Food Item	1,200 Cal	1,500 Cal	1,800 Cal
Breakfast	old-fashioned cooked oatmeal	½ cup	½ cup	½ cup
	fresh fruit cup	¾ cup	¾ cup	¾ cup
	skim milk or nonfat yogurt	8 oz	8 oz	8 oz
	decaf coffee or tea	as desired	as desired	as desired
	skim milk or light nondairy creamer	2 oz	2 oz	2 oz
		1 oz	1 oz	1 oz
Lunch	whole-grain bread	1 slice	1 slice	2 slices
	low-sodium ham or roasted turkey breast	2 oz	2 oz	3 oz
		2 oz	2 oz	3 oz
	with lettuce	as desired	as desired	as desired
	with salsa	1 tbs	1 tbs	1 tbs
	MARINATED CUCUMBERS TRICOLORE	½ cup	½ cup	½ cup
	strawberries or apple juice	1¼ cups	1¼ cups	2½ cup
		4 oz	4 oz	8 oz

Meal	Food Item	1,200 Cal	1,500 Cal	1,800 Cal
	water or decaf diet beverage	as desired	as desired	as desired
Snack	APPLES 'N' OATS MUFFIN	1	1	1
	with peanut butter	1 tbs	2 tbs	2 tbs
	skim milk or nonfat yogurt	—	4 oz	8 oz
	water or decaf diet beverage	as desired	as desired	as desired
Dinner	SCALLOPS CACCIATORE	2 cups	2 cups	2 cups
	braised zucchini (see BRAISED LEEKS recipe)	½ cup	1 cup	1½ cups
	endive & romaine salad	3 cups	3 cups	3 cups
	with low-calorie dressing	2 tbs	2 tbs	2 tbs
	pear or orange	1 small	1 large	1 large
	water or decaf diet beverage	as desired	as desired	as desired
Snack	gelatin (sugar free)	1 cup	1 cup	1 cup
	light whipped topping (optional)	2 tbs	2 tbs	2 tbs
	skim milk or nonfat yogurt	4 oz	4 oz	4 oz
	water or decaf diet beverage	as desired	as desired	as desired

DAY 14

Meal	Food Item	1,200 Cal	1,500 Cal	1,800 Cal
Breakfast	whole-grain bread	1 slice	2 slices	2 slices
	egg (poached, boiled, or scrambled)	1 large	2 large	2 large
	margarine (diet)	1 tbs	1 tbs	1 tbs
	grapes	15 small	30 small	30 small
	or pear	1 small	1 large	1 large
	skim milk or nonfat yogurt	4 oz	8 oz	8 oz
	decaf coffee or tea	as desired	as desired	as desired
	skim milk or light nondairy creamer	2 oz 1 oz	2 oz 1 oz	2 oz 1 oz
Lunch	SOUTHERN-STYLE ONION SOUP	1 cup	1 cup	1 cup
	BACON & CHEESE MELT with whole-grain bread	2 slices	2 slices	2 slices
	with diet cheese	2 oz	2 oz	2 oz
	with low-sodium bacon	1 slice	1 slice	1 slice
	tossed green salad	3 cups	3 cups	3 cups
	with cherry tomatoes	2	2	2
	with low-calorie dressing	2 tbs	2 tbs	2 tbs

Meal	Food Item	1,200 Cal	1,500 Cal	1,800 Cal
	nectarine or baked apple with cinnamon	1 small	1 small	1 large
	water or decaf diet beverage	as desired	as desired	as desired
Snack	CREAMY LIGHT CUSTARD	½ cup	½ cup	½ cup
	water or decaf diet beverage	as desired	as desired	as desired
Dinner	EASY VEGETARIAN CHILI 'N' CHEESE	1 cup	1 cup	2 cups
	endive & romaine salad	3 cups	3 cups	3 cups
	with olives	—	5 large	5 large
	with low-calorie dressing	2 tbs	2 tbs	2 tbs
	strawberries	2½ cups	2½ cups	2½ cups
	or banana	1	1	1
	water or decaf diet beverage	as desired	as desired	as desired
Snack	skim milk or nonfat yogurt	8 oz	8 oz	8 oz
	water or decaf diet beverage	as desired	as desired	as desired

DAY 15

Meal	Food Item	1200 Cal	1500 Cal	1800 Cal
Breakfast	whole-grain bread	1 slice	1 slice	1 slice
	peanut butter	1 tbs	1 tbs	1 tbs
	or cheese, (Swiss, American, Monterey Jack, cheddar)	1 oz	1 oz	1 oz
	orange juice	4 oz	4 oz	8 oz
	or orange	1 small	1 small	1 large
	skim milk or nonfat yogurt	4 oz	8 oz	8 oz
	decaf coffee or tea	as desired	as desired	as desired
	skim milk or light nondairy creamer	2 oz / 1 oz	2 oz / 1 oz	2 oz / 1 oz
Lunch	CLUBHOUSE SANDWICH	1	1	1
	assorted raw vegetables with FREE GI DIP	2 cups / 2 tbs	2 cups / 2 tbs	2 cups / 2 tbs
	plums	2 small	2 small	2 small
	or orange	1 small	1 small	1 small
	water or decaf diet beverage	as desired	as desired	as desire
Snack	pistachios	15	15	15
	plums	2 small	2 small	2 small
	or apple	1 small	1 small	1 small
	water or decaf diet beverage	as desired	as desired	as desire

Meal	Food Item	1,200 Cal	1,500 Cal	1,800 Cal
Dinner	leftover VEGETARIAN CHILI 'N' CHEESE	1 cup	1½ cups	2 cups
	Ryvita Crisp Bread	—	3	3
	romaine & red cabbage salad with low-calorie dressing	3 cups	3 cups	3 cups
		2 tbs	2 tbs	2 tbs
	STEAMED GREEN BEANS	1 cup	1 cup	1½ cups
	with garlic & thyme	as desired	as desired	as desired
	with olive oil	1 tsp	1 tsp	2 tsp
	pear or baked apple with cinnamon	1 small	1 large	1 large
	water or decaf diet beverage	as desired	as desired	as desired
Snack	skim milk or nonfat yogurt	8 oz	8 oz	8 oz
	water or decaf diet beverage	as desired	as desired	as desired

DAY 16

Meal	Food Item	1,200 Cal	1,500 Cal	1,800 Cal
Breakfast	Extra Fiber All-Bran or Fiber One cereal	⅔ cup	⅔ cup	1⅓ cups
	peach or apple	1 small	1 small	1 small

Meal	Food Item	1,200 Cal	1,500 Cal	1,800 Cal
	skim milk or nonfat yogurt	8 oz	8 oz	8 oz
	decaf coffee or tea	as desired	as desired	as desired
	skim milk or light nondairy creamer	2 oz. 1 oz	2 oz 1 oz	2 oz 1 oz
Lunch	Campbell's Old Fashioned Vegetable Soup	1 cup	1 cup	1 cup
	whole-grain bread	1 slice	2 slices	2 slices
	roast beef	2 oz	3 oz	3 oz
	with lettuce	as desired	as desired	as desired
	with tomato	1 slice	1 slice	1 slice
	with mayonnaise (light), (optional)	1 tbs	1 tbs	1 tbs
	tossed green salad	3 cups	3 cups	3 cups
	with sunflower seeds	1 tbs	1 tbs	1 tbs
	with low-calorie dressing	2 tbs	2 tbs	2 tbs
	plums	2 small	2 small	2 small
	or apple	1 small	1 small	1 small
	water or decaf diet beverage	as desired	as desired	as desired
Snack	fat-free Frookies cookies	2	2	2
	fresh fruit cup or mixed berries	¾ cup	1½ cups	1½ cups
	water or decaf diet beverage	as desired	as desired	as desired

Meal	Food Item	1,200 Cal	1,500 Cal	1,800 Cal
Dinner	POACHED SOLE WITH FENNEL	6 oz	6 oz	8 oz
	parslied potato, boiled with skin	1 small	1 med	1 med
	imitation sour cream	2 tbs	2 tbs	2 tbs
	BRAISED CELERY & ZUCCHINI STRIPS	½ cup	½ cup	1½ cups
	tossed green salad	3 cups	3 cups	3 cups
	with low-calorie dressing	2 tbs	2 tbs	2 tbs
	fresh fruit cup or citrus sections	¾ cup	¾ cup	¾ cup
	skim milk or nonfat yogurt	—	4 oz	4 oz
	water or decaf diet beverage	as desired	as desired	as desired
Snack	gelatin (sugar-free)	1 cup	1 cup	1 cup
	light whipped topping (optional)	2 tbs	2 tbs	2 tbs
	skim milk or nonfat yogurt	4 oz	4 oz	8 oz
	water or decaf diet beverage	as desired	as desired	as desired

DAY 17

Meal	Food Item	1,200 Cal	1,500 Cal	1,800 Cal
Breakfast	whole-grain bread	1 slice	1 slice	1 slice
	low-sodium ham	1 oz	1 oz	2 oz
	or diet cheese	1 oz	1 oz	2 oz
	orange	1 large	1 large	1 large
	or grapefruit	1	1	1
	skim milk or nonfat yogurt	4 oz	4 oz	8 oz
	decaf coffee or tea	as desired	as desired	as desired
	skim milk	2 oz	2 oz	2 oz
	or light nondairy creamer	1 oz	1 oz	1 oz
Lunch	whole-grain bread	1 slice	2 slices	2 slices
	peanut butter	1 tbs	2 tbs	2 tbs
	with fruit butter or sugar-free jelly (optional)	1 tbs	1 tbs	1 tbs
	assorted raw vegetables	1 cup	2 cups	3 cups
	with FREE GI DIP	2 tbs	2 tbs	2 tbs
	cantaloupe	1 cup	1 cup	1 cup
	or pear	1 small	1 small	1 small
	water or decaf diet beverage	as desired	as desired	as desired
Snack	BLUEBERRY OAT BRAN MUFFIN	1	1	1
	water or decaf diet beverage	as desired	as desired	as desired
Dinner	TURKEY ORIENTAL	2¼ cups	2¼ cups	2¼ cups

Meal	Food Item	1,200 Cal	1,500 Cal	1,800 Cal
	with bulgur or rice	⅔ cup	⅔ cup	1¼ cups
	tossed green salad	3 cups	3 cups	3 cups
	with olives	5 large	5 large	5 large
	or avocado	⅛	⅛	⅛
	with low-calorie dressing	2 tbs	2 tbs	2 tbs
	SCENTED PEACHES	1 small	1 large	1 large
	or Applesauce	½ cup	1 cup	1 cup
	water or decaf diet beverage	as desired	as desired	as desired
Snack	gelatin	1 cup	1 cup	1 cup
	with light whipped topping (optional)	2 tbs	2 tbs	2 tbs
	pistachios	—	—	15
	skim milk or nonfat yogurt	4 oz	8 oz	8 oz
	water or decaf diet beverage	as desired	as desired	as desired

DAY 18

Meal	Food Item	1,200 Cal	1,500 Cal	1,800 Cal
Breakfast	Ryvita Crisp Bread	3	3	3
	nonfat ricotta cheese	¼ cup	½ cup	½ cup

Meal	Food Item	1,200 Cal	1,500 Cal	1,800 Cal
	or 1% cottage cheese with cinnamon	¼ cup	½ cup	½ cup
	cantaloupe	1 cup	1 cup	1 cup
	or apple	1 small	1 small	1 small
	orange juice	—	4 oz	4 oz
	skim milk or nonfat yogurt	4 oz	4 oz	4 oz
	decaf coffee or tea	as desired	as desired	as desired
	skim milk	2 oz	2 oz	2 oz
	or light nondairy creamer	1 oz	1 oz	1 oz
Lunch	whole wheat pita pocket	1 small (1 oz)	1 small (1 oz)	1 large (2 oz)
	with low-sodium boiled ham	2 oz	2 oz	3 oz
	with shredded lettuce & alfalfa sprouts	1 cup	1 cup	2 cups
	with mayonnaise (light), (optional)	1 tbs	1 tbs	1 tbs
	tossed green salad	3 cups	3 cups	3 cups
	with tomato	1 large	1 large	1 large
	with sunflower seeds	2 tbs	2 tbs	2 tbs
	with low-calorie dressing	2 tbs	2 tbs	2 tbs
	low-sodium tomato juice or V-8	—	6 oz	6 oz

Meal	Food Item	1,200 Cal	1,500 Cal	1,800 Cal
	peach or apple	1 small	1 small	1 small
	water or decaf diet beverage	as desired	as desired	as desired
Snack	pumpernickel cocktail bread with light or whipped cream cheese	3 slices	3 slices	3 slices
	& dill	½ oz	½ oz	½ oz
	with cucumber	3 disks	3 disks	3 disks
	skim milk or nonfat yogurt	4 oz	4 oz	8 oz
	water or decaf diet beverage	as desired	as desired	as desired
Dinner	FUSILLI PESCATORE	1⅔ cups	1⅔ cups	1⅔ cups
	braised mushrooms (see BRAISED LEEKS recipe)	—	½ cup	1 cup
	tossed green salad	3 cups	3 cups	3 cups
	with olives	5 large	5 large	5 large
	with low-calorie dressing	2 tbs	2 tbs	2 tbs
	strawberries or fresh fruit cup	1¼ cups	1¼ cups	2½ cups
		¾ cup	¾ cup	1½ cups
	with light whipped topping (optional)	2 tbs	2 tbs	2 tbs
	water or decaf diet beverage	as desired	as desired	as desired

Meal	Food Item	1,200 Cal	1,500 Cal	1,800 Cal
Snack	graham cracker squares	3	6	6
	with fruit butter or sugar-free jelly (optional)	3 tsp	4 tsp	4 tsp
	FRUIT FRAPPE	½ cup	½ cup	½ cup

DAY 19

Meal	Food Item	1,200 Cal	1,500 Cal	1,800 Cal
Breakfast	whole-grain bread	1 slice	1 slice	1 slice
	peanut butter	1 tbs	1 tbs	1 tbs
	or cheese (Swiss, American, Monterey Jack, cheddar)	1 oz	1 oz	1 oz
	plums	2 small	4 small	4 small
	or pear	1 small	1 large	1 large
	skim milk or nonfat yogurt	8 oz	8 oz	8 oz
	decaf coffee or tea	as desired	as desired	as desired
	skim milk or light nondairy creamer	1 oz	1 oz	1 oz
Lunch	whole-grain bread	1 slice	2 slices	2 slices
	roasted turkey breast	2 oz	2 oz	2 oz

Meal	Food Item	1,200 Cal	1,500 Cal	1,800 Cal
	with lettuce	as desired	as desired	as desired
	with tomato	1 slice	1 slice	1 slice
	with mayonnaise (light), (optional)	1 tbs	1 tbs	1 tbs
	assorted raw vegetables	1 cup	1 cup	2 cups
	with FREE GI DIP	2 tbs	2 tbs	2 tbs
	fresh fruit cup	¾ cup	¾ cup	¾ cup
	water or decaf diet beverage	as desired	as desired	as desired
Snack	graham cracker squares	3	3	4
	with light or whipped cream cheese	½ oz	1 oz	1½ oz
	with fruit butter or sugar-free jelly (optional)	3 tsp	3 tsp	4 tsp
	pistachios	15	15	15
	peach or apple	1 small	1 small	1 large
	water or decaf diet beverage	as desired	as desired	as desired
Dinner	MOM'S LENTIL SOUP	1 cup	1 cup	1 cup
	whole-grain bread	1 slice	1 slice	1 slice
	BEEF CANCUN	⅔ cup	1 cup	1⅓ cups
	tossed green salad	3 cups	3 cups	3 cups
	with tomato	1 large	1 large	1 large
	with low-calorie dressing	2 tbs	2 tbs	2 tbs

Meal	Food Item	1,200 Cal	1,500 Cal	1,800 Cal
	pear or orange	1 small	1 small	1 small
	water or decaf diet beverage	as desired	as desired	as desired
Snack	graham cracker squares	—	—	3
	gelatin	1 cup	1 cup	1 cup
	light whipped topping (optional)	2 tbs	2 tbs	2 tbs
	skim milk or nonfat yogurt	4 oz	8 oz	8 oz
	water or decaf diet beverage	as desired	as desired	as desired

DAY 20

Meal	Food Item	1,200 Cal	1,500 Cal	1,800 Cal
Breakfast	old-fashioned cooked oatmeal	½ cup	½ cup	1 cup
	SCENTED PEACHES	1 small	1 small	1 small
	or applesauce	½ cup	½ cup	½ cup
	orange juice	—	4 oz	4 oz
	or grapefruit	—	½	½
	skim milk or nonfat yogurt	4 oz	8 oz	8 oz
	decaf coffee or tea	as desired	as desired	as desired
	skim milk or light nondairy creamer	2 oz	2 oz	2 oz
		1 oz	1 oz	1 oz

Meal	Food Item	1,200 Cal	1,500 Cal	1,800 Cal
Lunch	Ryvita Crisp Bread	3 slices	3 slices	3 slices
	leftover LENTIL SOUP	1 cup	1 cup	1 cup
	grated Parmesan cheese	1 tbs	1 tbs	1 tbs
	tossed green salad	3 cups	3 cups	3 cups
	with sunflower seeds	—	1 tbs	1 tbs
	with low-calorie dressing	2 tbs	2 tbs	2 tbs
	pear or orange	1 small	1 small	1 small
	skim milk or nonfat yogurt	4 oz	4 oz	4 oz
	water or decaf diet beverage	as desired	as desired	as desired
Snack	diet cheese	2 oz	3 oz	3 oz
	apple or pear	1 small	1 small	1 large
	water or decaf diet beverage	as desired	as desired	as desired
Dinner	COUSCOUS PILAF	⅔ cup	1 cup	1 cup
	CHICKEN AUX HERBES	1 drumstick	1 drumstick	2 drumsticks
	STEAMED ASPARAGUS or GREEN BEANS	1½ cups	2 cups	2 cups
	with lemon & garlic	as desired	as desired	as desired
	with olive oil	1 tbs	1 tbs	1 tbs
	endive & romaine salad	3 cups	3 cups	3 cups
	with low-calorie dressing	2 tbs	2 tbs	2 tbs

Meal	Food Item	1,200 Cal	1,500 Cal	1,800 Cal
	WHIPPED APPLE MERINGUE with light whipped topping (optional)	1 cup	1 cup	1 cup
		2 tbs	2 tbs	2 tbs
	water or decaf diet beverage	as desired	as desired	as desired
Snack	skim milk or nonfat yogurt	4 oz	4 oz	8 oz
	water or decaf diet beverage	as desired	as desired	as desired

DAY 21

Meal	Food Item	1,200 Cal	1,500 Cal	1,800 Cal
Breakfast	whole-grain bread	1 slice	1 slice	2 slices
	egg, poached, boiled, or scrambled	1 large	1 large	1 large
	margarine (light)	1 tbs	2 tbs	2 tbs
	orange juice or grapefruit juice	4 oz	4 oz	4 oz
	fresh fruit cup	¾ cup	¾ cup	¾ cup
	skim milk or nonfat yogurt	4 oz	8 oz	8 oz
	decaf coffee or tea	as desired	as desired	as desired
	skim milk or light nondairy creamer	2 oz	2 oz	2 oz
		1 oz	1 oz	1 oz

Meal	Food Item	1,200 Cal	1,500 Cal	1,800 Cal
Lunch	grilled cheese: with whole-grain bread	2 slices	2 slices	2 slices
	with diet cheese	2 oz	3 oz	3 oz
	with margarine (diet)	1 tbs	1 tbs	2 tbs
	roasted pepper strips	½ cup	1 cup	1 cup
	plums	2 small	2 large	2 large
	or orange	1 small	1 large	1 large
	water or decaf diet beverage	as desired	as desired	as desired
Snack	skim milk or nonfat yogurt	4 oz	4 oz	8 oz
	water or decaf diet beverage	as desired	as desired	as desired
Dinner	ORIENTAL STEAK SLICES	3 cups	3 cups	4 cups
	tossed green salad	3 cups	3 cups	3 cups
	with low-calorie dressing	2 tbs	2 tbs	2 tbs
	low-sodium tomato juice or V-8	—	—	6 oz
	mixed berries or fresh fruit cup	¾ cup	¾ cup	¾ cup
	with light whipped topping (optional)	2 tbs	2 tbs	2 tbs
	water or decaf diet beverage	as desired	as desired	as desired

Meal	Food Item	1,200 Cal	1,500 Cal	1,800 Cal
Snack	graham cracker squares	—	3	3
	gelatin with light whipped topping (optional)	1 cup	1 cup	1 cup
		2 tbs	2 tbs	2 tbs
	strawberries	1¼ cups	1¼ cups	1¼ cups
	or orange	1 small	1 small	1 small
	skim milk or nonfat yogurt	4 oz	4 oz	8 oz
	water or decaf diet beverage	as desired	as desired	as desired

CHAPTER SIX

The G-Index Diet Recipes

The following recipes, which are designed to be used with the G-Index Diet menus, have been divided into the following eight categories:

- Salad dressings and dips
- Sandwich spreads
- Muffins and grains
- Soups
- Egg dishes
- Entrees
- Vegetables
- Fruits

Each of these recipes has been created with an eye to keeping the Glycemic Index of the dish as low as possible, while at the same time providing the proper scientific nutritional balance.

SALAD DRESSINGS AND DIPS

The following are recipes for salad dressings and vegetable dips that are triple-good for you:

1. They are low GI foods.
2. They are easy to make and can be made in quantity in advance.
3. They are low in calories and a specified amount can be considered a "free" food, or one that contains fewer than 20 calories a portion.

YOGURT-DILL DRESSING

Yield: 1 cup. Free Portion: 2 tablespoons

1 cup plain nonfat yogurt
2 tablespoons fresh lemon juice
2 garlic cloves, minced
1 teaspoon chopped, fresh dill, or ¼ teaspoon dried
¼ teaspoon ground cumin

Whisk together all ingredients in a small bowl. Keep refrigerated in a covered container. Serve chilled.

CREAMY HERB DRESSING

Yield: 1 cup. Free Portion: 1 tablespoon

1 cup mayonnaise (light)
2 teaspoons fresh lemon juice or white wine vinegar
1 tablespoon finely chopped fresh parsley
1 tablespoon finely chopped fresh or frozen chives
2 teaspoons finely chopped fresh tarragon, or ¼ teaspoon dried

Whisk together all ingredients in a small bowl. Keep refrigerated in a covered container. Serve chilled.

BALSAMIC HERB DRESSING

Yield:' 1½ cups. Free Portion: as desired

1 cup balsamic vinegar
1 teaspoon Dijon-style mustard
¼ cup (5 sprigs) fresh parsley, finely chopped
¼ cup finely chopped fresh or frozen chives
1 teaspoon finely chopped fresh tarragon,
  or ¼ teaspoon dried
¼ teaspoon salt
⅛ teaspoon pepper

Whisk together all ingredients in a small bowl. Keep refrigerated in a covered container. Shake well before serving.

TOMATO AND HERB DRESSING

Yield: 1¼ cups. Free Portion: 1½ tablespoons

1 cup catsup
¼ cup red wine vinegar
1½ teaspoons dehydrated salad dressing mix, such as
  Knorr Herb & Onion or Good Seasons Italian

Whisk together all ingredients in a small mixing bowl. Keep refrigerated in a covered container. Shake well before serving.

HOT 'N' SPICY DRESSING

Yield: 1¼ cups. Free Portion: 3 tablespoons

1 cup Chunky Salsa, medium or hot, such as Frito Lay, Hot Chacha, or Old El Paso
¼ cup red wine vinegar

Whisk together all ingredients in a small mixing bowl. Keep refrigerated in a covered container. Shake well before serving.

SOUR CREAM AND CHIVE DIP

Yield: 1¼ cups. Free Portion: 1½ tablespoons

1 cup imitation sour cream
¼ cup fresh or frozen chives, finely chopped
Salt and pepper to taste

Whisk together the ingredients in a small mixing bowl. Keep refrigerated in a covered container. Serve chilled.

TANGY DILL DIP

Yield: 1¼ cups. Free Portion: 4 tablespoons

1 cup plain nonfat yogurt
¼ cup finely chopped fresh parsley
1 teaspoon finely chopped fresh dill, or ¼ teaspoon dried
1–2 garlic cloves, minced
Salt and pepper to taste

Whisk together all ingredients in a small mixing bowl. Keep refrigerated in a covered container. Serve chilled.

HOT 'N' CREAMY DIP

Yield: 1½ cups. Free Portion: 2 tablespoons

1 cup imitation sour cream
½ cup Frito Lay Chunky Salsa, hot

Whisk together the sour cream and salsa. Keep refrigerated in a covered container. Serve chilled.

SAVORY YOGURT DIP

Yield: 1 cup. Free Portion: 2 tablespoons

1 cup plain nonfat yogurt
1 ounce blue cheese, crumbled
1 garlic clove, minced
¼ cup grated onion, or ¼ teaspoon onion powder

Whisk together all ingredients in a small mixing bowl. Keep refrigerated in a covered container. Serve chilled.

HERBED COTTAGE CHEESE DIP

Yield: 1 cup. Free Portion: 3 Tablespoons

1 cup 1 percent cottage cheese
1 tablespoon imitation sour cream
1 garlic clove, minced
2 teaspoons finely chopped fresh dill, or ½ teaspoon
  dried
2 teaspoons finely chopped fresh tarragon, or ½
  teaspoon dried
Salt and pepper to taste

Whisk together all ingredients in a small bowl. Keep refrigerated in a covered container. Serve chilled.

SANDWICH SPREADS

HUMMUS-TAHINI SPREAD

Yield: 12 servings, approximately ¼ cup each

⅓ cup commercial tahini, such as from Cedar's
  Mediterranean Foods, Inc.
¼ cup lemon juice
2 cloves garlic, minced
¼ cup cold water
1 can (15 oz) chickpeas, rinsed and drained
3 tablespoons cold water

1. TO MAKE TAHINI SAUCE: Place first four ingredients in a blender and blend well (15–20 seconds).

2. Add chickpeas and water to tahini sauce; blenderize again for 20–30 seconds until the mixture is a smooth and creamy puree. Serve cold.

3. Paprika and chopped parsley may be added as optional garnishes.

4. May be stored, tightly covered in the refrigerator for up to two weeks. Layers may form during storage. Mix well before spreading.

1 serving: 113 calories, 12.1 g CHO, 5.8 g PRO, 5.3 g FAT, 0.0 mg CHOL

LIGHTNING ALTERNATIVE: Use two tablespoons per serving of a commercially prepared Hummus-Tahini Dip such as Cedar's Mediterranean Foods, Inc. *Note:* the commercial brand contains more fat and calories than ours. Therefore, the serving size for the Lightning Alternative is reduced from ¼ cup (4 tbs) to 2 tbs.

SPICY CHEESE DIP

Yield: 5 servings, ¼ cup each

1 cup soft white cheese (cottage, farmer, nonfat ricotta)
¼ cup plain nonfat yogurt
2 teaspoons dehydrated salad dressing mix, such as Knorr Herb & Onion or Good Seasons Italian

Process all ingredients in a blender for 10 seconds. Place in a closed container and keep refrigerated.

1 serving: 46 calories, 2.8 g CHO, 6.6 g PRO, 0.7 g FAT, 2.2 mg CHOL

TASTY CRABMEAT SALAD

Yield: 1 serving, ½ cup

1 can 3 ounces crabmeat, water-packed (see Note)
½ cup diced celery (1 stalk)
1 tablespoon finely chopped green onion
2 tablespoons calorie-reduced mayonnaise

1. Drain the crabmeat well.
2. Combine all ingredients in a small mixing bowl. Use immediately or refrigerate.

Note: For a smoother spread, puree the ingredients in a food processor or blender for 10 seconds. Three ounces of water-packed tuna or fresh chicken breast meat can be substituted for crabmeat.

1 serving: 138 calories, 13.8 g CHO, 15.4 g PRO, 2.2 g FAT, 86 mg CHOL

SHORTCUT: Chop celery and green onion in a food processor.

MUFFINS AND GRAINS

APPLES 'N' OATS MUFFIN

12 muffins

1½ cups old-fashioned rolled oats
1 cup whole wheat flour
1⅓ tablespoons fructose (see Note)
2 teaspoons baking powder
1 teaspoon ground cinnamon
½ cup unsweetened apple juice
¼ cup skim milk
1 large egg
2 tablespoons canola or other vegetable oil
1 tablespoon vanilla extract
1 medium apple, peeled, cored, and diced

1. Preheat the oven to 400° F. Line a muffin tin with paper cups or coat with nonstick cooking spray.
2. In a small bowl combine dry ingredients. Set aside. In a large mixing bowl, mix the juice, milk, egg, oil, and vanilla. Stir in the apple pieces.
3. Add the flour mixture and mix until moistened. Do not overmix.
4. Fill the muffin tin about three-quarters full. Bake for about 20 minutes or until top is golden brown.

Note: ¼ cup granulated sugar may be substituted for fructose, although it is not preferred.

Per muffin: 96 calories, 14.6 g CHO, 2.8 g PRO, 3.3 g FAT, 18.2 mg CHOL

SHORTCUT: Double the recipe and freeze the extra muffins.

LIGHTNING ALTERNATIVE: For one serving, substitute 2 ounces Muffin-a-Day or other fructose- or fruit-based low-fat muffin.

BLUEBERRY OAT BRAN MUFFIN

12 muffins

1¼ cups whole wheat flour
1 cup oat bran
2 tablespoons fructose (see Note)
1 tablespoon baking powder
¾ cup skim milk
½ cup egg substitute, or 1 whole egg + 1 egg white, beaten
1 teaspoon vanilla extract
2 tablespoons vegetable oil
¼ cup chopped walnuts
1 cup blueberries, fresh or frozen

1. Preheat the oven to 425° F. Line a muffin tin with paper cups or coat with nonstick cooking spray.
2. Combine flour, oat bran, fructose, and baking powder in a mixing bowl. Add remaining ingredients except the walnuts and blueberries. Mix thoroughly. Gently fold in walnuts and blueberries.
3. Fill each cup about three-quarters full, and bake for 15 to 18 minutes, or until tops are golden brown.

Note: ½ cup granulated sugar may be substituted for fructose, although it is not preferred.

Per 1 muffin (with egg): 162 calories, 21 g CHO, 7.4 g PRO, 6.3 g FAT, 18 mg CHOL

1 muffin (egg subst.): 159 calories, 21.1 g CHO, 7.3 g PRO, 5.9 g FAT, 0.3 mg CHOL

LIGHTNING ALTERNATIVE: For one serving, use 2 ounces Muffin-a-Day or other fructose-based low-fat muffin.

COUSCOUS PILAF

4 servings, ⅓ cup each

1 teaspoon olive oil
1 small onion, finely chopped
1⅓ cups water
1 garlic clove, minced
1 low-sodium chicken bouillon cube
1 teaspoon chopped fresh sage, or ½ teaspoon dried
⅔ cup couscous (see Note)
2 tablespoons chopped fresh parsley

1. Heat the oil in a small saucepan over medium heat. Add the onion and sauté until soft.

2. Add the water, garlic, bouillon cube, and sage and bring to a boil. Add the couscous, reduce the heat, and simmer, covered, for approximately 5 minutes or until all the liquid is absorbed. Stir in the parsley and serve immediately.

Note: ⅔ cup of rice may replace couscous, but it is not preferred.

1 serving: 79 calories, 13.6 g CHO, 4.3 g PRO, 1.4 g FAT, 0.0 mg CHOL

SHORTCUT: Chop onion in a food processor. Use garlic powder instead of fresh garlic.

CURRIED COUSCOUS

6 servings, ⅓ cup each

1½ cups cold water
1 chicken bouillon cube
1 cup couscous (see Note)
1 teaspoon diet margarine
1 teaspoon curry powder

1. Bring the water to boil in a medium saucepan. Add the bouillon cube and stir until dissolved.
2. Add all the other ingredients to the pan. Mix well. Cover tightly, and cook over low heat for 5 minutes.
3. Let stand 2 to 3 minutes before serving.

Note: Rice may be substituted for couscous, although it is not preferred.

1 serving: 77 calories, 15.9 g CHO, 0.8 g PRO, 0.5 g FAT, 0.0mg CHOL

SOUPS

COUNTRY-STYLE MINESTRONE

8 servings, 1 cup each

1 tablespoon olive oil
1 small onion, thinly sliced
2 medium potatoes, peeled and diced
2 large carrots, scraped and diced

2 celery stalks, thinly sliced
2 small zucchini, thinly sliced
1 can (15½ ounces) kidney beans
¼ cup minced fresh basil, or 1 teaspoon dried
1 tablespoon chopped fresh oregano, or 1 teaspoon
  dried
Salt and pepper to taste

1. Heat the oil in a 3-quart saucepan and sauté the onions until soft. Add the potatoes, carrots, celery, and zucchini. Add about 8 cups of water, making sure to cover the vegetables.

2. Mix in the kidney beans, dried herbs if using, and seasonings. Bring to a boil, then reduce the heat, cover, and simmer for 20 to 25 minutes. If using fresh basil and oregano, add in the last 5 minutes of cooking. Serve hot or at room temperature.

1 serving: 104 calories, 18.1 g CHO, 4.5 g PRO, 2.0 g FAT, 0.0 mg CHOL

SHORTCUT: Chop the potatoes, carrots, celery, and zucchini in a food processor.

LIGHTNING ALTERNATIVE: For one serving, use one of the following commercial soups: Health Valley Real Italian Minestrone, 7.5 ounces; Pritikin Low-Sodium Minestrone, 10 ounces; Campbell's Home Cookin' Minestrone 8 ounces; or Progresso Zesty Minestrone, 6 ounces. The last two have high sodium content.

MOM'S LENTIL SOUP

12 servings, 1 cup each

1 pound lentils, rinsed and drained
8 cups beef broth
2 large onions, chopped
2 medium carrots, sliced
2 celery stalks, thinly sliced
1 garlic clove, minced
1 can (6 ounces) tomato paste
Freshly ground pepper (optional)

1. Combine all the ingredients in a large pot. Cover, bring to a boil, then simmer for 1 hour. Correct seasoning.
2. Serve warm or hot with 1 teaspoon Parmesan cheese.

1 serving: 86 calories, 17.8 g CHO, 4.7 g PRO, 0.1 g FAT, 0.0 mg CHOL

LIGHTNING ALTERNATIVE: For one serving, substitute with any of the following commercial soups: Health Valley Fat Free Lentil & Carrots, 7.5 ounces; Pritikin Lentil, 8 ounces; Campbell's Home Cookin' Hearty Lentil, 6 ounces; or Progresso Lentil, 6 ounces. The last two have high sodium content.

MOSTLY PEA SOUP

12 servings, 1 cup each

3 tablespoons canola oil or other vegetable oil
1 medium onion, finely chopped
8 cups water

1 pound dried split peas
2 celery stalks, finely chopped
2 large carrots, sliced
1 bay leaf
Salt and pepper to taste

1. Gently heat the oil in a 3-quart saucepan. Add the onion and sauté until soft.

2. Pour water into the saucepan and add the split peas. When the water boils, add the celery, carrots, and bay leaf. Season with salt and pepper.

3. Cover the saucepan and simmer for 1 hour. Stir occasionally to prevent sticking. Serve hot. Soup may be pureed in a food processor or blender and served as a thick puree.

1 serving: 171 calories, 26.0 g CHO, 9.7 g PRO, 4.5 g FAT, 0.0 mg CHOL

SHORTCUT: Add onion with the other vegetables instead of sautéing it. Add the oil just before serving and mix well.

LIGHTNING ALTERNATIVE: For one serving, use any of the following commercial canned split-pea soups: Health Valley Fat Free Split Pea & Carrots, 12 ounces; Pritikin Split Pea, 8 ounces; or Progresso Green Split Pea, 9.5 ounces. The last has a high sodium content.

SOUTHERN-STYLE ONION SOUP

7 servings, approximately 1 cup each

5 cups beef broth
½ cup port wine
4 medium onions, thinly sliced in rings

1 bay leaf
6 tablespoons grated Parmesan cheese

1. Combine the broth and wine in a 2-quart saucepan. Bring to a boil.

2. Add the onion rings and bay leaf and cover. Reduce heat and simmer for 30 minutes, stirring occasionally.

3. Pour soup into warmed bowls. Sprinkle grated cheese on top. Serve immediately.

1 serving: *81 calories, 7.9 g CHO, 3.6 g PRO, 1.8 g FAT, 3.6 mg CHOL*

LIGHTNING ALTERNATIVE: For one serving, use either of the following commercial canned onion soups: Health Valley Golden Onion, 8 ounces; or Campbell's French Onion, 8 ounces (high sodium content).

EGG DISHES

CREAMY LIGHT CUSTARD

4 servings, ½ cup each

1½ cups skim milk
2 eggs lightly beaten
4 teaspoons fructose (see Note)
1½ teaspoons vanilla extract
Ground nutmeg (optional)

1. Preheat the oven to 325° F. Gently heat the milk in the top of a double boiler over low heat until it almost boils.

2. In a small mixing bowl, whisk together the eggs, fructose, and vanilla. Gradually stir in the hot milk.

3. Pour the mixture into 4 ½-cup ramekins (custard cups). Sprinkle tops with nutmeg, if desired.

4. Set the ramekins in a deep pan and pour in hot water to within ½ inch of their tops.

5. Bake 50 to 60 minutes. The custard is cooked when a knife tip inserted in the center comes out clean.

6. Remove ramekins from the pan. Chill 2 hours before serving.

Note: ⅓ cup granulated sugar may be substituted for fructose, although it is not preferred.

1 serving: 86 calories, 8.8 g CHO, 6.3 g PRO, 2.7 g FAT, 108 mg CHOL

LIGHTNING ALTERNATIVE: For one serving, use the following commercial reduced-calorie pudding mix: Jell-O Sugar Free Pudding and Pie Filling Cook'n Serve, ½ cup.

DEVILED EGGS WITH TOFU

2 servings, 4 halves each

4 large eggs, hard cooked
3 ounces soft tofu, drained
1 tablespoon Dijon-style mustard
Dash of Tabasco
Salt and pepper to taste
1 teaspoon reduced-calorie mayonnaise
Chopped fresh parsley (optional)
Paprika (optional)

1. Remove shells from the eggs. Slice the eggs lengthwise in half. Remove the yolks and discard.

2. In a small bowl mash the tofu with a fork. Add the mustard, Tabasco, salt and pepper, and mayonnaise. Mix well.

3. Fill the egg whites with the mixture. Sprinkle parsley and paprika on top, if desired. Serve chilled.

1 serving: 72 calories, 1.3 g CHO, 10.8 g PRO, 2.3 g FAT, 0.0 mg CHOL

SCRAMBLED EGG WITH SALSA

1 serving, 1 large egg

1 large egg (see Note)
1 tablespoon skim milk
Salt and pepper to taste (optional)
1–2 tablespoons salsa, mild or hot

1. Whisk all the ingredients together in a small bowl.

2. Coat a small skillet with nonstick cooking spray and set it over low heat. Pour the egg mixture into the pan and cook until the eggs are set, stirring occasionally to prevent sticking. Do not overcook. Serve hot.

Note: ½ cup egg substitute can be used instead of the egg and milk.

1 serving (with egg): 90 calories, 0.6 g CHO, 6.7 g PRO, 5.7 g FAT, 213 mg CHOL
1 serving (egg subst.): 60 calories, 2.0 g CHO, 10.0 g PRO, 1.8 g FAT, 0.0 mg CHOL

ENTREES

BACON AND CHEESE MELT

1 serving

2 slices whole-grain bread
2 ounces diet cheese
2 thin slices ripe tomato
1 slice (1 ounce) crisp low-sodium bacon

1. Lightly toast the bread on one side only. (Place toast in pan under broiler to toast lightly on one side.) Place one tomato slice on each piece of bread. Lay the cheese on top of each tomato. Place ½ slice of bacon on top of each slice of cheese.
2. Grill the open-face sandwiches until the cheese melts.

1 serving: 292 calories, 33.6 g CHO, 26.4 g PRO, 5.3 g FAT, 15 mg CHOL

SHORTCUT: Toast bread in toaster. Form layers as above and melt in microwave oven.

BEEF CANCUN

8 servings, ⅔ cup each

1¼ pounds 90 percent lean ground beef
1 medium onion, chopped
8 ounces fresh mushrooms, sliced
1 large green bell pepper, chopped
1 cup salsa, mild or hot

1. Brown the meat in a large nonstick skillet over low to moderate heat until cooked and easily separated into small pieces with a fork. Drain off the liquid and discard.

2. Add the vegetables to the meat, mix thoroughly, and sauté the mixture over moderate heat for 2 to 3 minutes.

3. Add the salsa and mix in well. Cover and simmer for 10 minutes. Serve hot.

1 serving: 121 calories, 7.8 g CHO, 18.0 g PRO, 2.4 g FAT, 52.6 mg CHOL

SHORTCUT: Chop onion and pepper together in a food processor. Use pre-sliced fresh mushrooms, available in some supermarket produce departments.

BREAST OF CHICKEN ROSEMARY

4 servings, approximately 3 ounces each

1 pound skinless, boneless chicken breasts, cut in half lengthwise
1 tablespoon olive oil
3 tablespoons dry white wine
4 tablespoons fresh lemon juice
2 sprigs fresh rosemary, or 1 tablespoon ground rosemary
Salt and pepper to taste (optional)

1. Preheat the broiler. Rinse and pat the chicken dry, then place it in a wide bowl.

2. In a small bowl whisk together the oil, wine, and lemon juice. Pour marinade over the chicken and turn once to coat both sides.

3. Coat a shallow baking pan with cooking spray and arrange chicken in a single layer.

4. Sprinkle the rosemary over the chicken. Add salt and pepper, if desired.

5. Broil the chicken 5 inches from the broiling unit for 20 minutes, turning once. Remove the chicken from the oven and let it stand covered for 5 minutes before slicing.

1 serving: 177 *calories,* 0.4 *g* CHO, 26.1 *g* PRO, 6.4 *g* FAT, 71.2 *mg* CHOL

CHEF'S SALAD

1 serving, approximately 2 cups

⅓ **cup julienned lettuce, rinsed and drained**
⅓ **cup julienned fresh spinach, rinsed and drained**
⅓ **cup canned kidney beans, rinsed and drained (for 1,800-calorie dieters only)**
1 cup chopped raw vegetables (broccoli, cauliflower, cucumber, green peppers, radishes, tomatoes, mushrooms, onions), in bite-size pieces, rinsed and drained
1 ounce roasted turkey breast, cut in strips
1 ounce Swiss cheese, cut in strips
2 tablespoons low-calorie salad dressing

1. In a large mixing bowl toss together the lettuce and spinach. Add the kidney beans (if applicable) and the remaining vegetables.

2. Top the salad with turkey strips and Swiss cheese.

3. Pour the dressing over the salad and toss well. Serve immediately.

1 serving: *167 calories, 7.0 g CHO, 15.7 g PRO, 8.5 g FAT, 35 mg CHOL*

SHORTCUT: Use pre-washed and pre-cut salad greens and vegetables. Layer the turkey and cheese on top of each other, roll up, and slice into strips.

CHICKEN AUX HERBES

8 servings, 1 drumstick each

1 tablespoon diet margarine
2 tablespoons chopped fresh parsley
1 tablespoon chopped fresh chives
2 teaspoons chopped fresh tarragon, or 1 teaspoon dried
Salt and pepper to taste (optional)
8 skinless chicken drumsticks

1. To prepare in a microwave oven (see Note), melt the margarine in a small plastic container. Stir in the herbs and seasonings.
2. Arrange the drumsticks in a shallow microwaveable casserole dish with the thickest part of the flesh facing outward. Brush the meat with half the melted herbed margarine.
3. Microwave at *medium-high* for 15 to 20 minutes. Turn the meat once halfway through the cooking and brush on the remaining margarine. Serve hot.

Note: If not using microwave, melt the margarine over low heat; stir in herbs and seasonings. Arrange the drumsticks in a preheated skillet that has been coated with nonstick cooking spray. Cook over low-medium heat for 25 to 30 minutes, turning several times.

1 serving: 101 calories, 0 CHO, 12.5 g PRO, 5.5 g FAT, 41 mg CHOL

SHORTCUT: Use dried parsley flakes and tarragon, and frozen diced chives. Soak drumsticks in salted water for 15 minutes for easy removal of skin.

CHICKEN CUTLETS LILLIAN

5 servings, approximately 2.5 ounces each

5 skinless chicken or turkey cutlets, approximately 3 ounces each
¼ cup skim milk
½ cup fresh bread crumbs
5 teaspoons olive oil

1. Preheat the broiler. Pound the cutlets until flat and dip them in the milk.
2. Coat the cutlets evenly with bread crumbs and arrange them in a shallow pan that has been coated with nonstick cooking spray.
3. Drizzle the oil evenly over the cutlets and broil about 5 inches from the heat for 5 to 6 minutes on each side. The cutlets should be nicely browned and crisp.

Note: Two tablespoons of warmed, sugar-free meatless tomato sauce can be poured over each cutlet just at serving.

1 serving: 186 calories, 7.5 g CHO, 20.8 g PRO, 7.2 g FAT, 54 mg CHOL

CHICKEN WITH MARKET VEGETABLES

3 servings, approximately 1½ cups each

1 tablespoon olive oil
1 pound skinless, boneless chicken breasts, cubed
2 garlic cloves, minced
½ cup chopped green onions
2 cups sliced fresh mushrooms
2 cups zucchini, sliced diagonally (see Note)
1 tablespoon lemon juice
Freshly ground pepper to taste (optional)
1 tablespoon chopped fresh parsley

1. Heat the olive oil in a large nonstick skillet over medium heat and sauté the chicken cubes for 3 minutes. Remove the chicken from skillet with a slotted spoon.

2. In the same skillet, sauté the garlic and vegetables for 2 minutes. Add the lemon juice and pepper. Stir thoroughly.

3. Return the chicken to the skillet and mix well with the vegetables. Cover and simmer for 5 minutes. Remove to a large platter and serve hot, sprinkled with parsley.

Note: If desired, substitute 2 cups fresh asparagus or broccoli.

1 serving: 251 calories, 8.8 g CHO, 34.8 g PRO, 8.3 g FAT, 85.2 mg CHOL

SHORTCUT: Ask your butcher for cubed breast meat. You can find pre-sliced fresh mushrooms and pre-squeezed lemon juice in many supermarket produce departments. Substitute garlic powder and dried parsley flakes to taste.

CLUBHOUSE SANDWICH

1 serving

2 slices whole-grain toast
1 tablespoon reduced-calorie mayonnaise
2 leaves lettuce
2 thin slices ripe tomato
2–3 ounces roasted chicken breast (see Note)
1 slice crisp bacon

1. Thinly coat both slices of toast with mayonnaise.
2. Between toast slices, form layers as follows: 1 lettuce leaf, 1 tomato slice, chicken breast, remaining tomato slice, crumbled bits of bacon, and remaining lettuce leaf.
3. Cut sandwich in half. Serve with 2 spears of dill pickle.

Note: For 1,200-calorie and 1,500-calorie menus, use 2 ounces chicken; for 1,800-calorie menu, use 3 ounces chicken.

1 serving (2 ounces chicken): 242 calories, 30.3 g CHO, 20.9 g PRO, 4.7 g FAT, 42.9 mg CHOL
1 serving (3 ounces chicken): 286 calories, 30.3 g CHO, 28.6 g PRO, 5.9 g FAT, 64.3 mg CHOL

EASY VEGETARIAN CHILI 'N' CHEESE

10 servings, 1 cup each

2 medium onions, chopped
3–4 garlic cloves, minced
1 can (29 ounces) crushed tomatoes
1 can (15 ounces) tomato puree

2 tablespoons chili powder
1 teaspoon red or white wine vinegar
½ teaspoon dried oregano
½ teaspoon dried basil
Freshly ground pepper to taste (optional)
3 whole dried hot red peppers (optional)
2 cans (16 ounces each) kidney beans, drained
10 ounces cheddar cheese, cut in strips

1. Coat a large skillet with nonstick cooking spray and set it over low heat. Add the onions and garlic and cook until soft.

2. Add the remaining ingredients except the beans and cheese. Simmer, covered, for 30 minutes, stirring occasionally.

3. Add the beans, mix well, and simmer 10 minutes longer, then add the cheese and heat through for 3 to 5 minutes. Serve hot.

1 serving: 231 calories, 23.5 g CHO, 13.8 g PRO, 10.0 g FAT, 30.0 mg CHOL

SHORTCUT: Chop onions in food processor. Use garlic powder and commercially shredded cheese.

LIGHTNING ALTERNATIVE: For one serving, use one of the following commercial chili entrees: Old El Paso Chili & Beans, 7.5 ounces; Health Valley Fat-Free Vegetarian Chili with Beans, 8 ounces; or Nile Spice Vegetarian Chili 'n Beans, 8.0 ounces; Burritos Low Fat Chili, 8.0 ounces; Fantastic Cha-Cha Chili, 8.0 ounces.

FILLET OF COD MILKY WAY

5 servings, approximately 4 ounces each

1½ pounds fresh cod fillets
¼ cup skim milk
½ cup fresh bread crumbs
Salt and pepper to taste (optional)
4 tablespoons diet margarine, melted
5 lemon slices

1. Preheat the broiler. Rinse and dry the cod fillets. Dip them in milk.
2. Coat the fillets evenly with bread crumbs and arrange in a shallow pan that has been coated with nonstick cooking spray. Add salt and pepper, if desired.
3. Drizzle the melted margarine over the fillets and broil about 5 inches from the heat for 4 to 5 minutes. Turn once; the bread crumbs should be nicely browned.
4. Serve immediately with lemon garnish (5 slices).

1 serving: 174 calories, 9.0 g CHO, *25.7 g* PRO, *3.2 g* FAT, *72 mg* CHOL

SHORTCUT: Use commercial plain bread crumbs.

FUSILLI PESCATORE

8 servings, 1⅔ cups each

2⅔ tablespoons olive oil
12 ounces (4 cups) fresh broccoli florets
1 can (28 ounces) crushed tomatoes with puree
1–2 garlic cloves, minced

Salt and pepper to taste
1 pound shrimp, washed and deveined
7 ounces (3 cups) corkscrew pasta (fusilli)

1. Heat the oil in a large skillet over moderate heat. Add the broccoli, tomatoes, garlic, and seasonings and simmer for 2 to 3 minutes.
2. Stir in the shrimp. Simmer, covered, for 2 minutes, stirring once. Remove the sauce from the heat. The shrimp should be pink and opaque in the center.
3. Cook the pasta in a large pot of boiling water according to package directions. When done, drain well and add to the shrimp sauce in the skillet. Toss well. Serve immediately.

1 serving: 228 calories, 29.2 g CHO, 17.2 g PRO, 5.7 g FAT, 83.7 mg CHOL

SHORTCUT: Use pre-cut fresh broccoli florets, available in most supermarket produce departments. Use garlic powder.

LIGHTNING ALTERNATIVE: For one serving, substitute Meatballs Parmigiana (see page 159) and 1 cup cooked spaghetti.

GREEN LASAGNA

12 servings, approximately 8½ ounces each

8 ounces lasagna noodles (12 strips)
1 teaspoon canola oil
1 tablespoon olive oil
1 medium onion, chopped
1 garlic clove, minced
1 pound part-skim ricotta cheese

4 tablespoons grated Parmesan cheese
1 package (10 ounces) frozen chopped spinach, thawed
    and well drained
2 egg whites, lightly beaten, or ¼ cup egg substitute
Freshly ground pepper to taste (optional)
1 tablespoon dried parsley flakes
⅛ teaspoon grated nutmeg
6–7 cups homemade or commercial meatless, sugar-free
    tomato sauce
6 ounces part-skim mozzarella cheese, grated

1. Preheat the oven to 350° F. Cook the lasagna noodles in salted boiling water for 8 minutes. (Adding 1 teaspoon of oil to the water will prevent the noodles from sticking together.) When cooked, drain immediately and lay flat to cool.

2. Heat the olive oil in a small skillet over medium heat and sauté the onion and garlic until softened. Set aside.

3. Combine the remaining ingredients except the tomato sauce and mozzarella in a large bowl. Add the sautéed onion and garlic and mix well.

4. Coat a 9 × 13 × 2-inch pan with nonstick cooking spray and spread ¼ cup tomato sauce over the bottom of the pan. Place 3 strips of lasagna, slightly overlapping, on the bottom of the pan. Spread one-fourth of the spinach-cheese mixture over the noodles and sprinkle with one-fourth of the grated mozzarella; cover with 1 cup of tomato sauce. Repeat the sequence with three more layers, ending with tomato sauce.

5. Cover the pan with foil and bake for 40 minutes. Uncover and continue baking another 10 to 15 minutes. Remove from the oven and allow to set for 5 minutes before cutting.

1 serving: 252 calories, 31.7 g CHO, 14.7 g PRO, 7.9 g FAT, 21.7 mg CHOL

SHORTCUT: Use 8 sheets of commercial precooked lasagna noodles, such as Ondine lasagne. Use garlic powder and pre-shredded mozzarella cheese.

LIGHTNING ALTERNATIVE: For one serving, use any of the following commercial frozen lasagna entrees: Lean Cuisine Lasagna with Meat & Sauce, 10.25 ounces; Healthy Choice Lasagna with Meat Sauce, 9 ounces; Budget Gourmet Light & Healthy Lasagna with Meat Sauce, 10 ounces; or Weight Watchers Lasagna with Meat Sauce, 11 ounces.

LIGHT MACARONI AND CHEESE

2 servings, 1½ cups each

1 package (7–8 ounces) macaroni and cheese mixture
⅓ cup imitation sour cream
¼ cup skim milk

1. Prepare the noodles according to package directions. Do not salt the water.
2. When cooked, drain the noodles thoroughly. Add the imitation sour cream and milk. Mix.
3. Add the packet of cheese sauce. Mix thoroughly. Serve immediately.

1½ cups: 443 calories, 70.3 g CHO, 16.5 g PRO, 12.2 g FAT 18.9 mg CHOL

MARINATED LONDON BROIL

9 servings, approximately 2 ounces each

For the marinade:
2 tablespoons olive oil
3 tablespoons red wine vinegar
½ cup dry red wine
3 garlic cloves, minced
3 tablespoons minced fresh parsley
1 tablespoon chopped fresh oregano, or 1 teaspoon
   dried
1 bay leaf
½ teaspoon freshly ground black pepper (optional)

1½ pounds top round or eye round London broil

1. In a small mixing bowl whisk together all the ingredients except the meat.

2. Place the steak in a deep bowl, pour on the marinade, and turn once to coat both sides. Cover and refrigerate for at least 4 hours, preferably overnight.

3. Preheat the broiler or prepare a charcoal grill. Broil or grill the meat for about 5 minutes on each side, or until done to taste.

4. Cut meat into thin diagonal slices across the grain. Serve warm or cold.

1 serving: 160.8 calories, trace CHO, *14.0 g* PRO, *10.0 g* FAT, *52 mg* CHOL

SHORTCUT: Use garlic powder, dried parsley flakes, and dried oregano.

LIGHTNING ALTERNATIVE: Do not marinate. Sprinkle with vinegar and herbs before cooking, and broil as above.

MEATBALLS PARMIGIANA

9 servings (18 meatballs), approximately 2.5 ounces each

1 pound 90 percent lean ground beef, turkey, or mixture of both
1 cup fresh bread crumbs
½ cup grated Parmesan cheese
3 tablespoons minced fresh parsley
1 garlic clove, minced
½ cup skim milk
4 egg whites, or ½ cup egg substitute
Salt and pepper to taste (optional)
2 cups sugar-free tomato sauce

1. Preheat the oven to 350° F. In a large bowl mix all the ingredients except the tomato sauce, and form into 18 meatballs (approximately the size of a golf ball).

2. Arrange the meatballs in a shallow pan and bake in the oven for 15 to 20 minutes, turning once. Remove from the oven and drain on paper towels.

3. Heat the tomato sauce in a large saucepan and add the meatballs.

4. Cook over low heat for 10 minutes. Serve over spaghetti (counted in meals of the day).

1 serving: 187 calories, 9.0 g CHO, 18.4 g PRO, 7.2 g FAT, 55 mg CHOL

SHORTCUT: Use commercial plain bread crumbs, dried parsley flakes, and garlic powder. This recipe produces a large yield; store leftovers in the freezer.

LIGHTNING ALTERNATIVE: For one serving, grill, bake, or broil 3 ounces of 90 percent lean ground beef, turkey, or mixture until done. Sprinkle with seasoned pepper or barbecue herbs.

ORIENTAL STEAK SLICES

6 servings, approximately 3 cups each

2 tablespoons olive oil
1 pound flank steak, cut diagonally into thin slices
2 cups fresh snow peas
2 cups thickly sliced fresh mushrooms
3–4 medium leeks, white part only, chopped
1–2 garlic cloves, minced
¼ cup dry red wine
6 ounces cholesterol-free "egg" noodles

1. Heat the oil in a large skillet over medium heat and sauté the flank steak until lightly browned.
2. Stir in the vegetables and cook about 5 minutes, until vegetables are crisp-tender. Add the wine and cook, covered, for 1 to 2 minutes. Remove from heat.
3. Cook the noodles according to the package directions. Drain well and transfer to a large serving bowl. Toss with the vegetable-meat mixture. Serve hot.

1 serving: 293 calories, 26.6 g CHO, 24.8 g PRO, 8.6 g FAT, 51.3 mg CHOL

SHORTCUT: Ask your butcher for flank steak strips. You can find pre-sliced fresh mushrooms in your supermarket produce department. Chop the leeks in a food processor. Use garlic powder.

PASTA PRIMAVERA

6 servings, 2 cups each

1 pound fresh broccoli florets, cut into bite-size pieces
1 pound zucchini, cut into thin diagonal slices
1 pound fresh mushrooms, sliced thin
1 pint (8 ounces) cherry tomatoes, cut in half
2 tablespoons olive oil
2 garlic cloves, minced
Salt and pepper to taste (optional)
½ pound thin spaghetti
2 tablespoons grated Parmesan cheese
12 leaves fresh basil, cut into strips

1. Steam the broccoli florets over boiling water until crisp-tender. Set aside. Rinse and drain the remaining vegetables.

2. Heat 1 tablespoon of the olive oil in a large skillet and lightly sauté the garlic. Add the zucchini and mushrooms; cook, covered, over low heat for 5 minutes. Add the steamed broccoli, tomatoes, and salt and pepper if desired. Mix well, and cook 2 minutes longer.

3. Cook the spaghetti in a large pot of boiling water according to package directions. When done, drain well and return the pasta to the pot.

4. Stir in the remaining tablespoon of olive oil and 1 to 2 tablespoons of water. Add the vegetables and grated Parmesan. Toss well and garnish with fresh basil strips. Serve hot or warm.

1 serving: 235 calories, 35.8 g CHO, 9.8 g PRO, 6.2 g FAT, 1.3 mg CHOL

SHORTCUT: You can find pre-cut broccoli florets and pre-sliced mushrooms in many supermarket produce departments. Use garlic powder.

POACHED SOLE WITH FENNEL

4 servings, approximately 4 ounces each

1¼ pounds fresh or frozen fillets of sole
1 tablespoon lemon juice
2 tablespoons dry white wine
1 teaspoon fennel seeds, crushed
Salt and freshly ground pepper to taste

1. Rinse the fillets and pat dry between paper towels. If using frozen fillets, make sure they are completely defrosted.
2. Place the fish in a large heated skillet that has been coated with nonstick cooking spray. Add the lemon juice, wine, and seasonings.
3. Cover and steam the fish over moderate heat for 6 to 8 minutes, or until it flakes easily when tested with a fork. Do not overcook. Serve immediately.

1 serving: 81 calories, 1 g CHO, 17.1 g PRO, 0.6 g FAT, 57 mg CHOL

SAUTÉED SCALLOPS MEDITERRANEAN

4 servings, approximately 4 ounces each

1¼ pounds fresh sea scallops*
4 canned plum tomatoes
1 tablespoon olive oil
¼ cup dry white wine
2 tablespoons fresh basil, or 1 teaspoon dried
Freshly ground pepper to taste

1. Rinse the scallops or shrimp and pat dry with paper toweling. Set aside.

2. Drain the tomatoes, cut them lengthwise in 1-inch strips, and remove all seeds. Reserve.

3. Heat the oil in a large skillet and brown the scallops or shrimp over high heat for 1 minute. Stir frequently to prevent sticking.

4. Add the wine, the reserved tomatoes, and the basil. Continue to cook over high heat for another minute. Stir to coat evenly. Season with freshly ground pepper.

*An equal amount of shrimp may be substituted for the scallops.

1 serving: 146 calories, 6.5 g CHO, 17.9 g PRO, 3.7 g FAT, 40 mg CHOL

SCALLOPS CACCIATORE

5 servings, approximately 2 cups each

1½ pounds fresh bay scallops
1 medium onion, finely chopped
1 green bell pepper, finely chopped
1 can (16 ounces) peeled tomatoes, drained and sliced
2 garlic cloves, minced
1 bay leaf
8 ounces spaghetti
Freshly ground pepper to taste (optional)
1 tablespoon chopped fresh parsley

1. Rinse scallops and drain well. Heat a large skillet that has been coated with nonstick cooking spray, add the scallops, and then add all the other ingredients except the spaghetti, pepper, and parsley. Cook over low heat for approximately 5 minutes, or until the scallops are thoroughly cooked, stirring occasionally.

2. Cook the spaghetti in a large pot of boiling water according to package directions. When done, drain well and arrange on a large serving platter. Pour the scallop sauce over the pasta, add the pepper, if desired, and mix well. Garnish with parsley. Serve immediately.

1 serving: 390 calories, 57.7 g CHO, 35.0 g PRO, 1.3 g FAT, 59.5 mg CHOL

SHORTCUT: The onion and pepper can be chopped together in a food processor. Use garlic powder and dried parsley flakes.

SESAME CHICKEN KABOBS WITH COUSCOUS

4 servings, approximately 3 ounces each

**1 pound skinless, boneless chicken breast,
 cut into 1-inch cubes
3 tablespoons light soy sauce
2 tablespoons olive oil
6 tablespoons dry white wine
1–2 garlic cloves, minced
2–3 tablespoons sesame seeds, lightly toasted
⅔ cup couscous (see Note)**

1. Rinse the chicken cubes and pat dry with paper toweling. Set aside in a bowl.

2. In a small bowl whisk together the soy sauce, olive oil, wine, and garlic. Pour over the chicken and marinate in the refrigerator for at least 30 minutes.

3. Preheat the grill or broiler. Skewer the chicken pieces loosely and broil, basting frequently with the marinade, for 5 to 8 minutes. When the chicken is done, roll it in sesame seeds.

4. While the chicken is cooking, prepare the couscous according to package directions.

5. Serve the chicken over hot couscous. Heat any remaining marinade to boiling and serve on the side (optional).

Note: Rice may be substituted for the couscous, although not preferred.

1 serving: 228 calories, 2.1 g CHO, 27.1 g PRO, 9.8 g FAT, 70.6 mg CHOL

SHORTCUT: Ask your butcher for cubed breast meat, or look for it in your supermarket meat department. Keep a jar of the marinade labeled in your refrigerator and use when needed.

TURKEY ORIENTAL

4 servings, approximately 2¼ cups each

2 tablespoons Worcestershire sauce
1 tablespoon low-sodium soy sauce
1 tablespoon dry red wine
4 teaspoons olive oil
¼ cup sliced green onions
1–2 garlic cloves, minced
8 cups chopped fresh vegetables, in bite-size pieces
 (see Note)
1 pound skinless, boneless turkey breast, cut into thin
 2-inch strips

1. Combine the sauces and wine in a small bowl. Set aside.

2. In a wok or large skillet, heat the oil over medium heat and sauté the green onions and garlic until softened.

3. Add the cut-up vegetables and stir-fry for 1 minute.

4. Add the reserved sauce mixture and turkey strips to the skillet. Cover and simmer for 2 to 3 minutes, or until the turkey is cooked through. Serve immediately over couscous or rice.

Note: Any combination of asparagus, green beans, broccoli, Brussels sprouts, cauliflower, eggplant, mushrooms, snow peas, green peppers, or zucchini may be used.

1 serving: 247 calories, 19.7 g CHO, 26.9 g PRO, 7.1 g FAT, 41.4 gm CHOL

SHORTCUT: Use garlic powder. You can find pre-cut fresh bite-size vegetables in your supermarket produce department. Use turkey tenders, or fillets, already cut in strips or ask your butcher for them.

VEGETABLES

BRAISED LEEKS

4 servings, 2 leeks each

8 medium leeks (see Note)
1 cup chicken broth
4 teaspoons diet margarine
Salt and pepper

1. Cut the leeks across the top, removing the rough green portion. Leave the white end intact. Wash the leeks thoroughly, carefully removing all dirt and sand between the leaves.

2. Steam the leeks in the chicken broth until tender, approximately 10 minutes. Drain.

3. Melt the margarine in the skillet over low heat. Add the leeks and cook 5 to 7 minutes, turning them often.

Note: Four cups of raw asparagus, broccoli, Brussels sprouts, eggplant, mushrooms, okra, snow peas, rutabaga, turnips, or zucchini can be substituted for leeks. Adjust cooking time accordingly.

1 serving: 65 calories, 6.0 g CHO, 1.4 g PRO, 4.3 g FAT, 0 mg CHOL

SHORTCUT: Serve the leeks steamed and drizzled with melted margarine.

MARINATED CUCUMBERS TRICOLORE

6 servings, ½ cup each

½ cup imitation sour cream
1 tablespoon red wine vinegar
2 teaspoons fructose (see Note)
2 teaspoons chopped fresh chives, or 1 teaspoon dried
2 teaspoons dill seed
Freshly ground pepper
1 medium red (Bermuda) onion, thinly sliced
1 medium cucumber, peeled and thinly sliced

1. Combine the first 6 ingredients in a medium mixing bowl.

2. Add the onion and cucumber. Toss to coat evenly. Transfer to a plastic container and marinate in the refrigerator at least 30 minutes before serving.

Note: Three tablespoons table sugar can be substituted for fructose, although it is not preferred.

1 serving: 25 calories, 2.5 g CHO, 0.6 g PRO, 1.2 g FAT, 0 mg CHOL

LIGHTNING ALTERNATIVE: For one serving, mix 1 medium cucumber and 1 small red onion, sprinkle with 2 tablespoons low-calorie dressing and ½ teaspoon oregano, and toss.

RATATOUILLE

10 servings, ½ cup each

2 tablespoons olive oil
1 large garlic clove, minced
2 medium onions, thickly sliced
1 small eggplant (8 ounces), cubed
1 large green bell pepper, sliced in 1-inch strips
2 small zucchini, thickly sliced
1 can (8 ounces) tomatoes, cut lengthwise in 1-inch strips, with liquid
¼ teaspoon dried thyme
¼ teaspoon dried oregano
1 tablespoon minced fresh basil, or ¼ teaspoon dried
¼ teaspoon freshly ground pepper
1 tablespoon chopped fresh parsley

1. Heat the oil in a 2-quart saucepan. Add the garlic and onions, and cook over moderate heat until the onions are soft. Add the eggplant, pepper, and zucchini and continue to cook for 5 minutes, stirring frequently.

2. Stir in the tomatoes and their liquid. Cover, reduce heat, and simmer for 20 minutes. Stir often to prevent sticking.

3. Add the remaining ingredients and mix well. Cook, uncovered, 5 more minutes, stirring often. Serve hot or cold.

1 serving: 72 calories, 8.4 g CHO, 0.7 g PRO, 4.3 g FAT, 0 mg CHOL

WILTED BOK CHOY

6 servings, 1 cup each

½ **large head bok choy (Chinese cabbage)**
1 **large garlic clove, minced**
1 **teaspoon fresh dill, or ½ teaspoon dried**
½ **teaspoon salt**
½ **teaspoon freshly ground pepper**

1. Shred the bok choy very fine, using a sharp knife. Rinse and drain well.

2. Steam the bok choy about 5 minutes, until tender.

3. Place in a serving bowl. Add garlic, dill, salt, and pepper. Mix well. Serve hot.

1 serving: 16 calories, 2.6 g CHO, 2.4 g PRO, 0 g FAT, 0 mg CHOL

"Generic" Low GI Vegetable Side Dishes

Vegetables are an integral part of any healthy, balanced diet, and the G-Index diet is no exception. In our twenty-one menus, vegetables—raw and/or cooked—are standard fare for lunch and dinner. Listed below are standardized recipes that allow you to create your own vegetable combinations without diverting far from the intended caloric allotment.

1 serving: 73 calories, 17.3 g CHO, 0.7 g PRO, 0.9 g FAT, 0 mg CHOL

ORIENTAL STIR-FRIED VEGETABLES

4 servings, 1 cup each

4 cups of any combination of peppers, cut in 1-inch strips
   Thickly sliced fresh mushrooms
   Thickly sliced onions
   Scallions, cut in ½-inch strips
   Snow peas
   Bamboo shoots
2 teaspoons vegetable oil
1½ tablespoons low-sodium soy sauce
1 tablespoon grated fresh ginger, or 1 teaspoon ground ginger
Salt to taste (optional)
1 tablespoon sesame seeds, toasted

1. Wash and drain the vegetables well. In a nonstick wok or skillet, heat the oil over high heat. Add vegetables and stir-fry for 2 minutes.
2. Add soy sauce and ginger, mix well, and stir-fry another

1 to 2 minutes; vegetables should be tender-crisp. Add salt if desired. Before serving, top with toasted sesame seeds.

1 serving: 54 calories, 5.0 g CHO, 1.7 g PRO, 3.6 g FAT, 0 mg CHOL

GRILLED VEGETABLES

4 servings, 1 cup each   2 VEGETABLE EXCHANGES

1 pound of raw eggplant or 3 pounds of raw zucchini or
** 1 pound of turnips, cut in ½ inch-thick slices**
1 tablespoon olive oil
¼ teaspoon dried oregano or thyme
Salt and pepper to taste

1. Preheat the broiler or prepare a charcoal grill. Wash and pat the vegetable dry with paper toweling. Do not peel it.
2. Lightly coat both sides of the vegetable slices with oil and sprinkle the oregano or thyme on the top only. Add salt and pepper as desired.
3. Broil or grill the vegetable 2 to 4 minutes on each side. Serve hot or cold.

1 serving: 58 calories, 6.5 g CHO, 1.4 g PRO, 3.6 g FAT, 0 g CHOL

BRAISED VEGETABLES

6 servings, ½ cup each

> 1 VEGETABLE EXCHANGE + ½ FAT EXCHANGE

4 cups of any of the following vegetables: asparagus, broccoli, Brussels sprouts, eggplant, mushrooms, okra, snow peas, rutabaga, turnips, zucchini
1 cup chicken or vegetable broth
4 teaspoons diet margarine
Salt and pepper to taste

1. Wash the vegetable and, if necessary, cut into appropriate-size pieces.
2. Steam the vegetable in the broth until almost tender. Drain.
3. Melt the margarine in a skillet over low heat. Add the vegetable and cook 3 to 7 minutes, turning often.

1 serving: 41 calories, 7.0 g CHO, 3.4 g PRO, 2.3 g FAT, 0.3 mg CHOL

STEAMED VEGETABLES

2 servings, 1 cup each   2 VEGETABLE EXCHANGES

4 cups of any of the following vegetables: artichokes, asparagus, broccoli, Brussels sprouts, cauliflower, eggplant, green beans, kohlrabi, leeks, mushrooms, okra, onions, snow peas, rutabaga, spinach, turnips, zucchini

1. Place a small amount of water on the bottom of a

steamer pot. Place the vegetable in the steamer basket, making sure it does not touch the water.

2. Bring water to a boil. Keep pot covered during cooking time. The time necessary to cook the vegetable to crisp-tenderness will depend on the size and cut of the vegetable.

1 serving: 44 calories, 9.8 g CHO, 4.2 g PRO, 0.4 g FAT, 0 mg CHOL

FRUITS

AMBROSIA

6 servings, ½ cup each

2 cups (orange and grapefruit) sections
2 medium red apples, cored and cut in bite-size cubes
½ teaspoon fructose (see Note)
1 teaspoon fresh lemon juice
½ banana, sliced
2 tablespoons shredded coconut

1. Place the citrus sections and apple cubes in a large mixing bowl. Sprinkle on the fructose and lemon juice, and mix thoroughly. Cover and refrigerate for 1 hour.

2. Just before serving, stir in the banana. Mix well.

3. Spoon into 6 individual dessert dishes. Sprinkle the coconut on top of the fruit. Serve immediately.

Note: 2 teaspoons table sugar can be substituted for fructose, although it is not preferred.

1 serving: 73 calories, 17.3 g CHO, 0.7 g PRO, 0.9 g FAT, 0 mg CHOL

SHORTCUT: You can find jars of pre-sectioned citrus fruits in the refrigerated juice section in your supermarket. Use bottled lemon juice from your supermarket produce department.

FRUIT FRAPPE

2 servings, ½ *cup*

8 ounces skim milk, plain nonfat yogurt, or fruited nonfat yogurt with artificial sweetener
1¼ cups fresh strawberries; or a small pear, orange, apple, or peach, or ½ banana, or ¾ cup fresh or frozen blueberries
Ground cinnamon

1. In a processor, puree the milk or yogurt and the fruit at high speed until frothy, at least 30 seconds.
2. Pour into a tall glass and sprinkle cinnamon on top. Serve immediately. Add crushed ice to glass if desired.

1 serving: 71 calories, 12.5 g CHO, 4.8 g PRO, 0.6 g FAT, 2 mg CHOL

SHORTCUT: Use pre-cut frozen fruit.

SCENTED PEACHES

4 servings, 1 whole peach each

4 ripe, medium peaches, halved and pitted
1 teaspoon fructose (see Note)
Dash of ground cinnamon
Pinch of nutmeg (optional)

1. Peel and quarter peaches. (Blanch the peaches for easy skin removal. Drop the halved, pitted peaches in boiling water for 2 minutes; run under cold water and peel back skin with a knife.) Place in a square pan with 1 inch of boiling water.

2. Sprinkle on the fructose, cinnamon, and nutmeg, if desired. Cover and simmer until tender, approximately 10 minutes. May be served warm or at room temperature.

Note: 4 teaspoons table sugar can be substituted for fructose, although it is not preferred.

1 serving: 49 calories, 12.7 g CHO, 0.6 g PRO, 0.1 g FAT, 0 mg CHOL

WHIPPED APPLE MERINGUE

2 servings, approximately 1 cup each

1 cup unsweetened applesauce or unsweetened stewed
**   fruit**
2 egg whites
1 tablespoon fructose (see Note)
Ground cinnamon, to taste

1. In a food processor or blender, puree the applesauce or fruit, egg whites, and fructose until the mixture is creamy and smooth.

2. Spoon into tall glasses. Sprinkle with cinnamon. Serve immediately.

Note: 4 tablespoons sugar can be substituted for fructose, but it is not preferred.

1 serving: *93 calories, 20.2 g* CHO, *3.6 g* PRO, *0.1 g* FAT, *0 mg* CHOL

LIGHTNING ALTERNATIVE: Use ½ cup unsweetened applesauce or stewed fruit plus ¼ ounce diet cheese (1 ounce equals no more than 55 calories) per serving.

CHAPTER SEVEN

The G-Index Shopping Lists and Other Useful Dieting Tools

This chapter is divided into three parts:

- The G-Index shopping lists, which have been coordinated to be used with each week of the G-Index Diet.
- A list of the specific foods and brand names recommended for those on the diet.
- Basic volume measurements and a conversion chart to help you determine exactly what portions you'll need for each food included in the diet.

Most likely, you'll want to refer back to this chapter as you shop and prepare your foods—especially when you're just beginning the diet. After you've been on the G-Index program for a few weeks, however, your knowledge of the foods and your sense of proper portion size will become automatic

SUGGESTED SHOPPING LISTS FOR EACH WEEK OF THE G-INDEX DIET

It's not necessary to buy all the foods listed here. In each day's menu, two or more options for certain food items have been suggested to allow for individual preferences and seasonal availability, such as for fruits, vegetables, and cheese. Simply refer to the menus, choose among the options provided, and cross off the shopping list those items you do not need or that you stock as a household staple.

WEEK ONE

CEREALS, GRAINS, PASTA, BREAD, CRACKERS

whole-grain bread
whole wheat pita bread
Extra Fiber All-Bran
Fiber One
old-fashioned rolled oats
Ry Krisp
graham crackers
linguine
spaghetti

MEAT, FISH, POULTRY, LEGUMES

London broil
90 percent lean ground beef, turkey, or mixture
scallops
cod fillets
skinless chicken or turkey breasts
roasted turkey breast
eggs
peanut butter (sugar-free)
split peas

DAIRY

hard cheese (Swiss, American, cheddar, Monterey Jack)
soft cheese (cottage, farmer, nonfat ricotta)
diet cheese
skim milk
nonfat yogurt (sugar-free)
Parmesan cheese

PRODUCE

Fruits

blueberries
cantaloupe
citrus sections
lemons
apples
pears
oranges
peaches
bananas
grapefruit

Vegetables

bell peppers
broccoli
asparagus
leeks
onions
celery
carrots
tomatoes
cucumbers
snow peas
pearl onions
green onions
potatoes

zucchini
eggplant
string beans
radishes
mushrooms
endive
romaine lettuce
iceberg lettuce

Spices

garlic
parsley
basil
rosemary

CANNED OR BOXED FOODS

white clam sauce (no sugar added, e.g., Progresso)
crabmeat
plum tomatoes
stewed tomatoes
tomato sauce (sugar-free)
chickpeas
kidney beans
macaroni and cheese
Cup-a-Soup (onion or chicken broth)
applesauce (unsweetened)
gelatin (sugar-free)
pea soup (Progresso, Health Valley, or Pritikin)

CONDIMENTS

apple or plum butter
light cream cheese
diet margarine
olive oil
vegetable oil

red wine vinegar
dry red wine
dry white wine
low-sodium or light soy sauce
low-calorie salad dressing
reduced-calorie mayonnaise
imitation sour cream

SEASONINGS AND HERBS (DRIED OR FRESH)

dehydrated salad dressing
chicken bouillon cubes (low sodium)
table sugar (fructose)
shredded coconut
oregano
bay leaves
basil
cumin
rosemary
thyme
salt and pepper

BEVERAGES

decaffeinated coffee
decaffeinated tea
decaffeinated diet soda
sparkling water or seltzer
grapefruit juice

MISCELLANEOUS

egg substitute
light nondairy creamer
low-calorie pudding mix
light whipped topping
sesame seeds
dry-roasted almonds

WEEK TWO

CEREALS, GRAINS, PASTA, BREAD, CRACKERS

whole-grain bread
whole wheat pita bread
All-Bran Extra Fiber
Fiber One
old-fashioned rolled oats
graham crackers
rice
couscous
lasagna noodles
thin spaghetti
spaghetti

MEAT, FISH, POULTRY, LEGUMES

peanut butter (sugar-free)
eggs
low-sodium boiled ham
roasted turkey breast
low-sodium bacon
skinless chicken breast
flank steak
bay scallops
(soft) tofu

DAIRY

hard cheese (Swiss, American, cheddar, Monterey Jack)
part-skim mozzarella
part-skim ricotta
diet cheese
grated Parmesan cheese
skim milk
nonfat yogurt (sugar-free)

CANNED OR BOXED FOODS

 tomato sauce (sugar-free)
 tomato puree
 peeled whole tomatoes
 crushed tomatoes
 water-packed tuna
 applesauce (unsweetened)
 gelatin (sugar-free)

PRODUCE

Fruits

 cantaloupe
 apples
 pears
 oranges
 lemons
 bananas
 grapes
 strawberries
 tangerines
 nectarines

Vegetables

 bell peppers
 broccoli
 asparagus
 yellow onion
 green onions
 Bermuda onion
 tomatoes
 cherry tomatoes
 zucchini
 mushrooms
 spinach
 endive
 romaine lettuce

bok choy
alfalfa sprouts
bean sprouts
cucumbers
sweet potatoes

Spices

garlic
parsley
basil
dill
chives

CONDIMENTS

apple or plum butter
light cream cheese
diet margarine
olive oil
canola or other vegetable oil
red wine vinegar
dry white wine
low-sodium or light soy sauce
low-calorie salad dressing
reduced-calorie mayonnaise
Dijon-style mustard
catsup
salsa
imitation sour cream

SEASONINGS AND HERBS

beef bouillon cubes (low sodium)
chicken bouillon cubes (low sodium)
fructose
Tabasco
nutmeg
cinnamon

vanilla extract
dried dill
dill seed
basil
oregano
curry
chili powder
chives
salt and pepper

BEVERAGES

decaffeinated coffee
decaffeinated tea
decaffeinated diet soda
sparkling water or seltzer
orange juice
apple juice

WEEK THREE

CEREALS, GRAINS, PASTA, BREAD, CRACKERS

whole-grain bread
whole wheat pita bread
pumpernickel cocktail bread
Ryvita Crispbread
Extra Fiber All-Bran
Fiber One
old-fashioned rolled oats
whole wheat flour
oat bran
couscous
rice
corkscrew pasta (fusilli)
cholesterol-free ''egg'' noodles
graham crackers
bulgur

MEAT, FISH, POULTRY, LEGUMES

peanut butter (sugar-free)
roasted chicken breast
roasted turkey breast
low-sodium boiled ham
bacon
roast beef
sole fillets
shrimp
90 percent lean ground beef
chicken drumsticks
flank steak
lentils

DAIRY

cheese (Swiss, American, Monterey Jack, cheddar)
diet cheese
grated Parmesan cheese
nonfat ricotta cheese
1 percent cottage cheese
eggs
skim milk
nonfat yogurt (sugar-free)

CANNED OR BOXED FOODS

Campbell's Old Fashioned Vegetable Soup (or Campbell's
    Healthy Request Vegetable Soup)
R. W. Frookie Cookies
gelatin (sugar-free)
applesauce (unsweetened)
low-sodium tomato juice
V-8 juice with no salt added
crushed tomatoes in puree
tomato paste

PRODUCE

Fruits

oranges
lemons
grapefruit
plums
pears
peaches
eating apples
baking apples, e.g. Rome Beauty
blueberries
raspberries
strawberries
cantaloupe
avocado

Vegetables

iceberg lettuce
romaine lettuce
endive
tomatoes
red cabbage
green beans
potatoes
celery
zucchini
green onions
asparagus
alfalfa sprouts
broccoli
Brussels sprouts
cauliflower
eggplant
mushrooms
snow peas
green peppers
cucumbers

turnips
onions
carrots
leeks

Spices

garlic
parsley
dill
chives

CONDIMENTS

reduced-calorie mayonnaise
low-calorie dressing
olive oil
vegetable oil
imitation sour cream
apple or plum butter
Worcestershire sauce
low-sodium or light soy sauce
light cream cheese
salsa
diet margarine
dry white wine
dry red wine

SEASONINGS AND HERBS

thyme
fennel seeds
tarragon
sage
vanilla extract
cinnamon
salt and pepper
chicken bouillon (low sodium)

BEVERAGES

decaffeinated coffee
decaffeinated tea
decaffeinated diet soda
sparkling water or seltzer
orange juice
apple juice

MISCELLANEOUS

egg substitute
light nondairy creamer
light whipped topping
pistachios
sunflower seeds
walnuts
large olives
baking powder

LIST OF SPECIFIC FOODS RECOMMENDED FOR THE DIET

The purpose of this list is to help you identify specific foods that are desirable for the G-Index Diet. Usually, this means that the foods are low in fat and low on the G-Index scale. This knowledge is particularly important for products such as breads, cereals, and diet cheeses, which are foods where the ingredients and processing of different brands may vary widely. One problem: many of the best choices are not sold nationally. This is particularly true of fresh breads, which are often made and sold locally.

You can have confidence in the foods on our lists. Other brands may be just as good, but are not included because we did not encounter them or could not test them. However, you should recognize that manufacturers of low G-Index foods may sell many similar products that are undesirable high G-Index foods. Our recommendation of a particular food would not ordinarily extend to related products of that manufacturer.

CEREALS

General Mills Fiber One
Kashi Breakfast Pilaf
Kellogg's Extra Fiber All-Bran
Old fashioned Quaker Oats or Mother's Oats oatmeal porridge
Kellogg's Fiberwise (formerly Heartwise)

DIET CHEESE (55 calories per ounce)

Alpine Lace Free 'n' Lean line including "American style" and Mozzarella
Borden—all cottage cheeses
Breakstone's—all cottage cheeses
Crowley—all ricotta cheeses, all cottage cheeses
Friendship—all cottage cheeses
Frigo—all ricotta cheeses
Laughing Cow Reduced Mini Cheese
Mini Bonbel Reduced Calorie Cheese
Lite-Line—all varieties of cheese product
Polly-O—all ricotta cheeses, Polly-O non-fat line
Sargento—pot cheese, all ricotta cheeses
Smart Beat American Sandwich slices
Weight Watchers—all cottage cheeses, creamed cheeses, all varieties of imitation cheese

Regular cheeses usually contain about 100 calories per ounce. Cheeses labeled "reduced calories" are required to have ⅓ fewer calories than the regular version. Other commonly used terms such as "diet" or "light" do not have a legal definition. Therefore, you must look at the calorie section of the label to find cheeses that meet our stricter standard of 55 calories per ounce or less. The specific brands on this list all meet that standard.

SALAD DRESSINGS (10 calories or less per tablespoon)

Estee Red Wine Vinegar, Creamy Dijon, Creamy Italian, Creamy French, Zesty Italian, Thousand Island, Bacon & Tomato, Blue Cheese, Creamy Garlic

Featherweight Zesty Tomato, Healthy Recipes Italian, Creamy Cucumber, Herb, Red Wine Vinegar, Russian

Good Seasons No Oil Italian

Hain No Oil Caesar, No Oil Garlic & Cheese, No Oil Herb, No Oil Italian

Kraft Free Italian, No Oil Italian

Newman's Own Light Italian

Pritikin Italian, Herb Vinaigrette, Garlic & Herb

Seven Seas Free Italian, Free Red Wine Vinegar

Weight Watchers Caesar Salad, Italian Style, French Style, Tomato Vinaigrette

Wish-Bone Lite Italian

Regular salad oils and dressings typically have 50 or more calories per tablespoon. Many low calorie dressings have 20–30 calories per tablespoon. A few have as few as 6 calories per tablespoon. The brands listed here contain 10 calories or less per tablespoon.

REDUCED-CALORIE (LIGHT) MAYONNAISE

Estee Reduced Calorie

Featherweight Reduced Calorie

Hellman's Light, Cholesterol Free

Kraft Light, Free

Kraft Miracle Whip Light, Free

Smart Beat Reduced Calorie

Weight Watchers Reduced Calorie, Cholesterol Free

LIGHT CREAM CHEESE

King Smoothee Imitation

Philadelphia Light Whipped

Weight Watchers

IMITATION SOUR CREAM

Breakstone Light Choice
Friendship Light Sour Cream
King Sour
Land O' Lakes Light
Light 'n' Lively Sour Cream Alternative

WHOLE-GRAIN OR STONEGROUND BREADS

Prefer brands that have as first ingredient whole, sprouted, or cracked grain. Next best choice is 100% stoneground bread, preferring coarser to finer ground.

Alvarado Farms 100% Sprouted Wheat Bread or Bagel
Arnold Stoneground 100% Whole Wheat
Braunschlagger European Style Rye
Brown Hill's Organic Sesame
Ezekiel Sprouted Grain Breads
Jane Parker 100% Whole Wheat
Martin's Dutch Country 100% Stoneground Whole Wheat
   Sandwich Roll
Matthew's All Natural Whole Wheat Bread
Old World Black Forest Bread
Orowheat Stoneground Whole Wheat Bread
Pepperidge Farm Sprouted Wheat
Pritikin Whole Grain Whole Wheat, Rye
Rudolph's Double Crust Schinkenbrot Whole Grain Rye
Shiloh Farms Cracked Wheat; 100% Whole Grain Wheat
Shra Lins Greek Style Whole Wheat Pita
Taystee 100% Stoneground Whole Wheat
Toufayan's 100% Whole Wheat Pita
Vermont Bread Company 100% Whole Wheat, Alfalfa
   Sprouts, Sprouted Wheat, Oat Bran Oatmeal, Whole
   Wheat Whole Grain, Whole Wheat Sourdough
Wild's Whole Grain Breads
Wonder Stoneground 100% Whole Wheat Bread

WHOLE-GRAIN OR STONEGROUND CRACKERS

ak-mak 100% Stoneground 'Whole of the Wheat Cracker'
Fiber Crisp
Finn Crisp Thin Crisp Bread
Goodman's 100% Stoneground Whole Wheat Matzoh
Kavli Crispbread
Ry Krisp
Ryvita Crisp Bread
Venous Par-ak Stoneground Whole Wheat Wafer Bread
Wasa Crispbread

BASIC MEASUREMENTS

VOLUME MEASUREMENTS

Pinch	=	$\frac{1}{16}$ teaspoon
Dash	=	$\frac{1}{8}$ teaspoon
3 teaspoons	=	1 tablespoon
2 tablespoons	=	$\frac{1}{8}$ cup or 1 fluid ounce
4 tablespoons	=	$\frac{1}{4}$ cup or 2 fluid ounces
5$\frac{1}{3}$ tablespoons	=	$\frac{1}{3}$ cup
8 tablespoons	=	$\frac{1}{2}$ cup or 4 fluid ounces
10$\frac{2}{3}$ tablespoons	=	$\frac{2}{3}$ cup
12 tablespoons	=	$\frac{3}{4}$ cup or 6 fluid ounces
16 tablespoons	=	1 cup or 8 fluid ounces
$\frac{1}{2}$ pint	=	1 cup
1 pint	=	2 cups or 16 fluid ounces
2 pints	=	4 cups or 1 quart
1 liter	=	1 quart plus 3 fluid ounces
4 quarts	=	1 gallon

CONVERSION CHART

LIQUID MEASURES

Fluid Ounces	U.S. Measures	Imperial Measures	Milliliters
	1 tsp.	1 tsp.	5
¼	2 tsp.	1 dessert spoon	7
½	1 T.	1 T.	15
1	2 T.	2 T.	28
2	¼ cup	4 T.	56
4	½ cup or ¼ pint		110
5		¼ pint or 1 gill	140
6	¾ cup		170
8	1 cup or ½ pint		225

SOLID MEASURES

U.S. and Imperial Measures		Metric Measures	
Ounces	Pounds	Grams	Kilos
1		28	
2		56	
3½		100	
4	¼	112	
5		140	
6		168	
8	½	225	

OVEN TEMPERATURE EQUIVALENTS

Fahrenheit	Gas Mark	Celsius	Heat of Oven
225	¼	107	Very Cool
250	½	121	Very Cool
275	1	135	Cool
300	2	148	Cool
325	3	163	Moderate
350	4	177	Moderate
375	5	190	Fairly Hot

9			250 (¼ liter)
10	1¼ cups	½ pint	280
12	1½ cups or ¾ pint		340
15		¾ pint	420
16	2 cups or 1 pint		450
18	2¼ cups		500 (½ liter)
20	2½ cups	1 pint	560
24	3 cups or 1½ pints		675
25		1¼ pints	700
27	3½ cups		750
30	3¾ cups	1½ pints	840
32	4 cups or 2 pints or 1 quart		900
35		1¾ pints	980
36	4½ cups		1000 (1 liter)

9		250	¼
12	¾	340	
16	1	450	
18		500	½
20	1¼	560	
24	1½	675	
27		750	¾
28	1¾	780	
32	2	900	
36	2¼	1000	1
40	2½	1100	
48	3	1350	
54		1500	1½

400	6	204	Fairly Hot
425	7	218	Hot
450	8	232	Very Hot
475	9	246	Very Hot

PART III

Designing Your Own
G-Index Diet

CHAPTER EIGHT

It's Time to Develop
Some Flexibility!

The fixed menus and recipes in Part II are your starting point. Now you're ready to make the G-Index Diet a way of life by learning to *design* your own program.

There are three fundamental factors that allow you to move from a fixed diet to the flexibility necessary for a lifetime eating plan. These include the following:

1. Tactics to protect you from hunger, including a workable approach to eating out. This chapter describes the main methods and suggests ways you can make them part of your approach to eating.
2. An ability to use simple foods and snacks that serve as "hunger stoppers" during the most vulnerable times of the day. Chapter Nine deals with this issue.
3. Building your own set of menus through the G-Index food exchange lists described in Chapter Eight.

Now let's turn to the first of these factors: tactics.

TACTICS TO PROTECT YOU FROM HUNGER

Every successful dieter needs a basic strategy and a set of tactics to put that strategy into practice. The strategy behind the G-Index Diet involves eating daily menus consisting largely of foods that are low on the Glycemic Index. You followed that strategy automatically with the fixed menus and recipes in Part I of this book. At that stage of the program, you didn't need to make strategy decisions about food because those decisions were made for you.

But eventually most people want to vary their menu beyond a particular twenty-one-day plan. They need to pick up a snack when they're on the run. They like to eat out in a restaurant, at least on occasion. How can you stay on the diet when you go off the fixed menus? The following tactics give you a strong foundation for developing the flexibility you need.

Tactic 1. *Eat low GI meals at breakfast and you'll consume fewer calories at lunch.* Scientific studies have shown that people who eat meals that are low to moderate on the Glycemic Index tend to feel more satisfied and thus eat smaller lunches. For example, eating a cereal like All-Bran, which has a moderate GI rating, holds off hunger better than high GI cereals like shredded wheat.

In one investigation, people who ate low GI cereals consumed 150 calories less by the end of lunch than those on high GI cereals. This means that in less than a month, a person eating a high GI breakfast might take in enough extra calories to add one pound to his or her body weight.

Tactic 2. *Eat low GI meals for dinner and you'll be more satisfied the next morning at breakfast.* Researchers have found that dinner foods that are low on the Glycemic Index— such as grapefruit, broccoli, or pasta—have a lasting impact through the night. When you wake up in the morning, the foods you eat for breakfast tend to raise your blood sugar and insulin less and stimulate your appetite less.

In a key 1988 study at the University of Toronto, conducted by Dr. Thomas Wolever and associates, the first group of participants ate low GI foods in the evening, including red lentils, pearled barley, skim cheese, and margarine. Another group of participants ate high GI dinners including instant potatoes, whole-meal bread, skim cheese, and margarine. Then the two groups ate the same high GI breakfasts the next morning.

The results indicated that blood sugar and insulin levels of those who had consumed the low GI meals the night before went up more slowly after breakfast than did the levels of participants who had eaten the high GI dinners. So what you eat for dinner the night before can exert a significant impact a half a day later on your blood sugar—and on your appetite.

Tactic 3. *Eat a given quantity of low GI foods in several sittings during the day instead of eating those same food quantities in fewer sittings.* Small, frequent feedings result in less insulin stimulation, no greater blood sugar elevation, and more satisfaction than when the same foods are eaten in three separate meals. Thus you can improve the Glycemic Index impact of your meals, *and* suppress your appetite, by consuming multiple small meals instead of the traditional "three squares" a day.

Tactic 4. *Lessen the appetite-stimulating effect of a high GI food by mixing it with low GI fare.* Mixing low GI foods and high GI fare in the same meal results in a composite or average Glycemic Index that is somewhere between the extremes, according to various investigations. So if you like a "bad" diet food with a high Glycemic Index, you can still eat some of it so long as you eat it with a low GI item. The mixture will reduce the tendency of the total meal to trigger hunger.

For example, you might eat spaghetti, which has a low GI, along with a little rice or bread, which has a high GI. The overall GI impact on your blood sugar and insulin is somewhere between each of the two sets of GI values.

Note: You should assume that this sort of "mixed" GI meal will average out mathematically according to the GI ranking of the foods and the amounts consumed in calories. So if you eat equal caloric amounts of one food ranked class 1 on our GI scale and another food ranked class 3, the resulting mixture is class 2—or in a desirable category on the G-Index.

Tactic 5. *Take in low GI, high-carbohydrate foods when you are about to engage in heavy physical activity or exercise.* Mounting evidence shows that a low GI pre-game meal may prolong endurance during strenuous exercise. For athletes, if you eat high carbohydrate meals, choose your carbohydrates with care. Pick ones that are low on the Glycemic Index, such as pasta, oranges, or grapefruit, and are thus consistent with the G-Index Diet.

Tactic 6. *Prepare yourself mentally to embark on the G-Index Diet.* The G-Index Diet has been designed to minimize any seesaw or yo-yo syndrome. But enhancing your motivation and deepening your commitment to the program can certainly help.

Knowing that more than nine out of ten people who lose weight on a diet put it right back on, a number of researchers are emphasizing the mental preparation necessary to stay on a diet. Dr. Kelly D. Brownell, a psychologist at Yale University, has discovered that success in dieting depends on the ability of the person to make a long-term commitment, manage stress, and pursue an exercise program.

Here are some questions that you might grapple with *before* embarking on the G-Index Diet. Also, ask the questions periodically *after* you've started the diet:

- Why do I want to diet? A short-term reason, such as losing weight to impress someone in whom you have a romantic interest or an old friend you haven't seen in a long time, isn't adequate. The reason should have some long-term or permanent ingredient, such as losing to increase energy, look younger, or reduce cardiovascular risk factors.
- What are the main pressures in my life—and how much do they preoccupy my thinking? If you're facing a major emotional challenge, such as a divorce, death of a loved one, or job change, this may not be the time to diet. You have to devote some thought and time to starting a new program, and it's also advisable to keep stress at a minimum as you're developing new food habits. After you've been on the G-Index Diet for a while—and after you've

experienced some success—the stresses you encounter will be less bothersome. In the beginning stages, though, it's helpful to avoid outside pressure and concentrate on the changes you're making in your life.

• Am I willing to incorporate some regular exercise in my life as I begin dieting? As I mentioned earlier, regular exercise is the best predictor of long-term success on a diet. Even a superior regimen such as the G-Index approach, which actually reduces hunger drives, will benefit from outside support such as exercise. But you *don't* have to kill yourself with an Olympic-level routine. Just walking a couple of miles a day, three to four times a week, is enough to enhance significantly your potential for success on the diet.

(You don't *have* to exercise on this diet, of course. Many people who have not been involved in a regular aerobic program have succeeded in taking off weight and keeping it off. But consistent exercise certainly helps, and I recommend such activity without qualification.)

Tactic 7. *Pick three to five of your favorite fruits or other snack foods that are low on the Glycemic Index, and store them in a handy place in your home or office.* We all get busy or preoccupied on occasion and forget to buy or prepare a proper snack. If hunger strikes in those moments, the temptation to eat anything within reach can be overwhelming. So be sure that an easy-to-eat G-Index diet food is close at hand.

For example, if you like grapefruit juice, pears, and apples, keep an ample supply handy at all times. The fructose sugar in these low GI foods ensure a slow rise in blood sugar and insulin. With these "safety net" foods on hand, you'll have the means to satisfy your appetite *and* stay on the diet. This technique will work if you feel fatigued or if you experience a food craving in the late afternoon, in the evening before bedtime, or at some other vulnerable moment.

Tactic 8. *Choose the right breakfast because that's your most important dieting decision for the day.* Good choices at breakfast promote consistent diet habits throughout the day. Bad choices at breakfast can be ruinous. Here's why. Blood sugar and insulin levels are relatively low in the morning because your stomach has emptied and your food is completely digested. Many breakfast foods are high in carbohydrate and low in fat—for instance, toast, bagels, and many hot or cold cereals. Since most breads and cereals are high GI foods, they tend to digest quickly and turn into glucose.

A lack of fat in many breakfasts allows these low GI items to cause an even greater surge in blood sugar. This occurs because one of the nutritional virtues of fat is to slow down the pace of digestion in the stomach. When there is little or no fat in the gastrointestinal tract, high G-Index carbohydrates rush from the intestines into the blood as though they were race cars heading toward a finish line. Blood sugar escalates, triggering insulin, which in turn stimulates the appetite.

Then, blood sugar falls to a low level and provokes an adrenaline discharge—the body's "shock" reaction that prevents hypoglycemia. The increase in adrenaline may result in nervous distress and a craving for sweets or other poor food choices.

A low GI breakfast presents quite a different picture. A selection of low GI breads, cereals, muffins, fruits, and low-fat milk products will prevent high blood sugar surges. These foods will replenish your body's sugar reserves (glycogen), which are depleted overnight. At the same time, low GI items will assure a slow, steady input of glucose into your bloodstream. This action provides you with stable blood sugar and insulin levels throughout the morning.

But some dieters object, "I'm hardly ever hungry when I wake up in the morning. Why not just skip breakfast and avoid all the trouble?"

It is true that when insulin levels are low, as happens after you've gone a while without food, hunger may be minimal. Insulin in the blood declines overnight, and the failure to put food in the stomach over a period of many hours keeps the insulin low and may actually suppress hunger in the morning. Many people don't become hungry until *after* they eat breakfast! (*Note:* Low insulin levels that occur during long fasts over several days or weeks are one reason that hunger strikers can go on for so long. They actually lose their appetite after a time.)

Despite some of the virtues of fasting, I urge people on the G-Index Diet to eat breakfast *even if they aren't hungry*. Skipping breakfast, or any other meal or snack, lowers the body's metabolic rate. When you eat, the body is triggered to "rev up" and burn more calories. Similarly, eating five or six times a day stimulates the fat-burning mechanism even more frequently and results in more weight loss than eating the same number of calories in two or three large meals. So skipping breakfast or any other scheduled meal is, quite literally, penny wise and pound foolish.

To help you in your planning, here are some generic suggestions for low GI breakfasts. These are presented with categories or types of foods, rather than as fixed menus, such as those that are included in Chapter Five. Here, you can just plug in the specific foods from the lists in Chapter Three. Also, you may need to consult the food exchange lists in Chapter Ten.

BREAKFAST 1 (cereal, fruit, milk)

Low GI hot or cold cereal (½ to 1 cup)

Low GI fruit, melon, or fruit juice

Skim milk or nonfat yogurt (8-ounce portion plain or fruited, with artificial sweetener)

Coffee or tea (preferably decaffeinated)

Optional light nondairy creamer (2 tablespoons)

BREAKFAST 2 (cheese, fruit, bread)

Low GI bread, graham crackers, or whole-grain Ry Krisp crackers

Cheese (Swiss, Cheddar, American, or Monterey Jack) (1 ounce); or diet cheese (55 calories to the ounce, 2 ounces)

Coffee or tea (preferably decaffeinated)

Optional light nondairy creamer (2 tablespoons)

BREAKFAST 3 (muffin, fruit, natural peanut butter)

Our low GI muffin (page 136)
Low GI melon or fruit
Natural peanut butter (1 tablespoon on muffin)
Low GI fruit
Coffee or tea (preferably decaffeinated)
Optional light nondairy creamer (2 tablespoons)

BREAKFAST 4 (egg, egg white, egg substitute)

Boiled or poached egg, or ½ cup egg substitute (scramble
it using nonstick vegetable spray), or two egg whites,
scrambled
For omelet, add 1 cup onions, pepper, herbs, salsa, preferred vegetables
Low GI bread or toast, or Ry Crisp whole-grain crackers
Fruit or fruit juice

Tactic 9. *Take maximum advantage of your dinner menu,
which requires deceptively easy diet decisions.* In some ways,
dinner should be the easiest meal of the day for a dieter. It's
usually eaten at home, so you have more control over what
you put on the table. The evening meal is usually the largest
meal of the day, with nearly half the day's calories (about 40
to 45 percent of the total daily intake of calories and fats).
There is ample opportunity to design interesting and filling
courses in accordance with G-Index principles.

Dinner typically contains more fat than other meals because
the evening repast includes more high-protein foods such as
fish, poultry, and red meat. Even on a low-fat diet, most fat
is consumed in the evening.

Fat slows the pace of digestion, reducing the blood sugar's
stimulating effect accompanying carbohydrate foods.

Even if you include some foods that are high on the G-
Index, you can lessen their effect by mixing them with low
GI items (see Tactic 4). For example, you may serve mostly
low GI dishes one evening. But you may also decide you'd
like to eat a baked potato (high GI) rather than a boiled potato

(low GI), or white bread (high GI) rather than whole-grain bread (low GI).

Such a meal will do considerably less damage to your blood sugar and insulin balance in the evening than if you eat the same high G-Index foods alone as a snack. For that matter, it's better to eat them at dinner rather than at lunch or breakfast, since the morning and noon meals typically contain fewer calories. This means that the high GI products automatically have a more significant impact on your sugar and insulin.

But don't overdo high GI foods with dinner. If you focus mainly on low GI choices at night, you'll have greater protection from the dieter's scourge, late-night snacks. And as you know from Tactic 2, low G-Index eating at dinner means more stable blood sugar and insulin the next morning.

In short, you can practically *ensure* permanent weight loss and maintenance with smart G-Index meal planning in the evening. Here are a few generic suggestions for evening meals to give you an idea about what's possible:

EVENING MEAL 1

Six ounces of fish, shellfish, poultry, or lean meat
Unlimited steamed vegetables
Salad with low-fat dressing
Boiled potato, pasta, or beans
1 tablespoon diet margarine or low-fat sour cream
Low-fat, low GI dessert

EVENING MEAL 2

2 cups pasta with shellfish sauce
Tossed green salad with low-calorie dressing
1 cup grilled vegetables
Small dish (3 ounces) low-fat frozen yogurt (artificially sweetened, no sugar added)

EVENING MEAL 3

1 cup lentil or split pea soup
6 ounces baked red snapper fillets

Tossed green salad with low-calorie dressing
1 cup steamed vegetables
Small (3 ounces) fresh fruit tart

EVENING MEAL 4

3 cups Oriental chicken and vegetable stir-fry
1 cup steamed rice
Small dish (3 ounces) of sorbet and fortune cookie

EVENING MEAL 5

Shrimp tostada
Tomato and onion salad with oil and vinegar
6 corn tortilla chips, with ½ cup salsa
¾ cup fresh low GI fruit salad

Tactic 10. *Be shrewd in your selection of restaurant lunches.* Many people who are on diets eat lunch at a restaurant because they work during the day. Unfortunately, restaurants aren't often sensitive to the dieter, and so people on a G-Index program have to pay particular attention to their midday selections. To help you plan lunches and other meals that you eat out, I've provided some guidelines.

The biggest challenges are to avoid the following:

- High G-Index breads, such as white and regular whole wheat.
- Hidden fat, which is contained in such products as mayonnaise and salad dressings, and is often mixed in salads with otherwise excellent, low-fat protein foods such as tuna and chicken.
- Excessive servings of any food, which many restaurants provide.

Lunch portions in restaurants and cafeterias tend to be large. Emotionally it's hard for many people to leave food on their plate. The food is so tempting! Or maybe they just can't screw up the courage to ask the waiter to bring a doggie bag. So following their mother's instructions, they clean their plates—and break their diets. Another problem is that you really don't have much control over the meal you're served. The cook will typically give you fatty cuts of beef and extraordinary quantities of butter or salad dressing unless you instruct otherwise.

Suggestions for Salad Bars

Heap your plate with green vegetables, mixed beans, cottage cheese, turkey or flaked tuna, and reduced-calorie dressing. This type of salad is available at most restaurants and even some fast-food places. (*Caution:* Regular salad dressings contain 45 to 50 calories per tablespoon. Creamy and blue cheese dressings can have 75 calories or more per tablespoon. Choose the low-calorie type, or consider bringing your own!)

Omit or at least limit the toppings that go on these salads, such as croutons, bacon bits, and sunflower seeds—all of which contain considerable amounts of fat and calories.

Chef's salads usually provide 6 ounces of ham, roast beef, or poultry. These contain 300 to 500 calories, so you'll do best by leaving off half the meat.

Suggestions for Chinese Food

Chinese food offers several decent GI choices provided you ask for steamed or lightly stir-fried selections, rather than those that are deep-fried, and you avoid the high-salt MSG. Most Chinese restaurants are happy to tailor your meal to give you less fat, fewer calories, and less salt. For example, you might choose steamed Chinese vegetables with shrimp or chicken; take the sauce on the side, and use it sparingly. Another choice is Egg Drop or hot and sour soup, or select steamed or stir-fried fish or chicken.

On the other hand, Chinese noodles, deep-fried dishes, and sweet-and-sour sauce may be high on the G-Index, high in fat, or both. Most forms of rice, when eaten by themselves, also have a fairly high GI. That's why you're often hungry an hour after a Chinese meal! But if you eat small to moderate servings of rice or any of these other items, along with large quantities of steamed greens and other low GI items, you'll enjoy a meal that is relatively low on the Glycemic Index, low in calories, and low in fat.

Suggestions for Dairy and Fruit Dishes

Endless combinations of fruit are usually available in restaurants and delis. For the G-Index Diet, you should emphasize cantaloupe and honeydew melon over pineapple and watermelon. The latter are high on the G-Index and trigger high blood sugar and insulin release.

Add protein by choosing cottage cheese, low-fat yogurt with a low GI, or low-fat milk.

Suggestions for Pizza

No pizza is a really terrific diet food, but there are far worse choices. Ironically, the high GI of the pizza crust is reduced by combining it with the relatively high-fat cheese. The secret here is portion control. You should limit yourself to one small slice, or two at the most. Also, choose a plain cheese or vegetable pizza over pepperoni, sausage, or other meat pizza.

A standard pizza slice topped with vegetables has about 165 calories and 8 grams of fat. If you watch your fat intake closely during the rest of the day, you can still keep your overall consumption low. The best idea, though, is to find a pizza place that offers a low-fat cheese topping or a pizza that is relatively dry, with minimal oil.

To keep the calories low and ensure you'll end up with a relatively low total GI for the meal, follow your pizza slice with a low-GI fruit, such as a pear, apple, or orange.

Suggestions for Lean Meat and Poultry

Many restaurants have special diet selections such as fresh broiled or grilled fish, broiled chicken, sliced white meat turkey, lean roast beef, or lean hamburger. Vegetables and fruit should be included, but size of the burger should be limited to 2 to 3 ounces, not ¼ pound. Also, avoid the french fries or potato chips that usually accompany the hamburger.

Stay away from tuna, chicken, or egg salads. These may be good choices for home eating, where you can oversee preparation. But in restaurants these dishes invariably contain about 4 tablespoons of regular mayonnaise (at 100 calories per tablespoon) in every 3 ounces of the salad.

Suggestions for Soups

The best soup choices are lentil, barley, bean, split pea, clear chicken broth, or clear beef broth. But restaurant soups are invariably high in salt, unless you make a special request for a low-salt type. So don't be surprised if you puff up a pound or two after one of these soups. It's only water that accumulates in your body as a result of the salt, and after a day of normal eating it will come right off.

Soups tend to be weak on protein, but that's no problem if you follow our overall guidelines; you'll get plenty of protein during the rest of the day. Or if you like, you can add protein *and* a low GI ingredient by having a glass of skim milk or a low GI yogurt with the soup.

Suggestions for Sandwiches

I enjoy quick-serve deli sandwiches, but there are some problems. Even if you order low-fat foods, such as turkey breast, roast chicken, or lean roast beef, the portions typically are too large for an effective diet. These sandwiches tend to contain a minimum of 6 ounces of meat or poultry. Also, you have to add a minimum of 200 calories for the bread (or more if you're getting a hero). With butter, mayonnaise, or salad dressing, you're looking at a minimum of 500 to 600 calories—with a fairly high G-Index to boot. At the least, avoid salami, cheese, oil, or Russian dressing on your sandwich.

Lean meat or poultry sandwiches are acceptable if you save about half for lunch tomorrow, or perhaps for a light supper; restrict the meat to 3 ounces; or use low G-Index bread, such as coarse pumpernickel.

THE G-INDEX EATING OUT PLAN

We've devised a comprehensive program to help you follow the G-Index Diet when you eat out at a restaurant. The first section is a summary set of suggestions to help you choose foods in different types of restaurants, including fast-food places. This should be useful for the occasional meal out. The second section offers more detailed guidelines, helpful for an extended trip or longer period away from home.

You'll note that this second section includes a number of items that may have to be purchased at a supermarket or deli. We're assuming that you may want to eat an occasional breakfast or snack in your hotel room or while you're on the run between appointments.

Also, precise measurements have been included for items in the second section. No one can be perfect in measuring amounts at a salad bar. The portions are just target quantities for each of the three diet levels.

Set aside ten or fifteen minutes some evening to practice visualizing how much of a given food is equal to 1 cup or 1 ounce. This way, you can learn to estimate how much you are being served.

The Summary Guide to Eating Out

You will do best if you take your choice from among these.

DINER

Breakfast
Cantaloupe and cottage cheese
Old-fashioned oatmeal
Plain omelet
Whole-grain cereal, berries, and skim milk

Lunch or Dinner
Cottage cheese salad platter
Flaked tuna salad platter
Vegetable omelet
Vegetable barley soup and whole-grain bread or crackers
Lentil soup and rice, whole-grain bread or crackers

AMERICAN

Business Lunch
Beef barley soup; lettuce, tomato, and egg salad
Manhattan clam chowder; tossed salad
Vegetarian chili
Chicken Caesar salad
Mushroom crepe
Grilled seafood platter
Shrimp cocktail and tossed green salad

Dinner
Poached white fish, parslied potatoes, green beans
Broiled chicken breast, clear sauce, salad, asparagus
Roast turkey platter, green salad, roasted potatoes
London broil, green salad, boiled new potatoes
Baked ham, sweet potato, applesauce

ITALIAN

Lunch
Minestrone; tomato, mozzarella, and basil salad
Polenta and grilled mushrooms
Roasted peppers, sun-dried tomatoes over pasta
Prosciutto, figs, or cantaloupe, tossed green salad
Sardines, garlic bread, tossed green salad

Dinner
Vegetable lasagna, salad, fruit
Vegetarian or cheese pizza, salad, fruit
Pasta and tomato or vegetable sauce, salad, fruit
Pasta and shellfish, salad, fruit
Spinach ravioli, salad, fruit
Rosemary chicken breast, zucchini, potatoes, fruit
Baked eggplant Parmesan

CHINESE

Lunch or Dinner
Steamed vegetables, rice, fruit
Stir-fried vegetables, rice, fruit
Chicken lo mein, rice, fruit
Mandarin chicken, rice, steamed vegetables, fruit
Stir-fried chicken and broccoli, rice, fruit
Chicken or shrimp stir-fry, rice, fruit

JAPANESE

Lunch or Dinner
Sashimi, stir-fried vegetables, rice, fruit
Sushi, stir-fried vegetables, fruit
Gyoza (chicken dumplings), steamed vegetables, fruit
Nabemono (casseroles), fruit
Chicken or turkey teriyaki, stir-fried vegetables, rice, fruit
Tofu dishes, steamed vegetables, noodles, fruit

AMERICAN COFFEE SHOP

Lunch
Chef's salad, whole-grain bread, fruit
Lemon-pepper chicken breast, cottage cheese, peaches
Marinated salmon, pumpernickel, grilled tomato, fruit
Sautéed scallops, tomato and onion salad, bread, fruit
Garden vegetable stir-fry, whole-grain bread, fruit

Dinner

Flank steak, corn, broccoli, salad, fruit
Grilled swordfish, bean salad, beets, fruit
Roasted Cornish hen, potatoes, cauliflower, fruit
Seafood kabobs, grilled vegetables, bread, fruit

MEXICAN

Lunch or Dinner

Bean corn tortilla, tomato and onion salad
Seviche (marinated fish), peppers, salad, papaya
Shrimp tostada, yellow squash, salad, fruit

DELI

Lunch

½ turkey sandwich on rye, fruit
Macaroni and beef, salad, fruit cup
½ lean roast beef sandwich, pickles, fruit

SUPERMARKET

Take-out Lunch

Salad bar (fruit, vegetables, flaked tuna, cottage cheese),
  whole-grain crackers, milk
Baked potato with vegetable or yogurt topping, fruit
Soups (vegetable-barley, minestrone, bean, lentil, tomato),
  whole-grain crackers, fruit, yogurt
Cottage cheese and fruit platter, whole-grain crackers, to-
  mato juice
Vegetable lasagna, fruit, milk or yogurt
Pasta primavera, fruit, milk or yogurt
Oriental vegetables, rice, fruit, milk or yogurt

FAST-FOOD SPOTS

The following is a list of food choices found in specified
eateries that, while they all may not be ideal because of fat

or sodium content, remain the best selections available. These choices should be kept in mind when designing the whole day's meals and snacks.

McDonald's
Apple Bran Muffin
McLean Deluxe
Chunky Chicken Salad
Small Hamburger

Wendy's
Baked Potato
Chili con Carne
Grilled Chicken Fillet
Junior Hamburger

Burger King
Chef Salad (no dressing)
Chunky Chicken Salad (no dressing)
Chicken Tenders
Small Hamburger

Taco Bell
Bean Burrito
Chicken Fajita
Frijoles and Cheese
Soft Taco
Tostada with Red Sauce
Beef Taco
Small Hamburger

Hardee's
Pancakes
Chicken Stix
Grilled Chicken Sandwich
Chicken & Pasta Salad
Small Hamburger

Roy Rogers
Salad bar—vegetables and fruit only
Roast Beef Sandwich
Small Hamburger

Dairy Queen
  Small Hamburger

Jack-in-the-Box
  Chicken Fajita Pita
  Club Pita Without Sauce

L. J. Silver
  Clam Chowder
  Corn on the Cob
  Seafood Salad

Pizza Hut
  Cheese Pan Pizza

Domino's
  Cheese Pizza
  Ham Pizza

SNACKS

TCBY
  Sugar-Free, Fat-Free Yogurt Cup
  Small Sugar-Free Smoothie
  Sugar-Free Vanilla Frozen Yogurt Bar, Sugar-Free Chocolate Coating
  Small Lite Bite Shake
  Small Lite Bite Fruit Smoothie

Baskin-Robbins
  Sugar-Free Jamoca Swiss Almond, 4-ounce cup
  Sugar-Free Strawberry, 4-ounce cup
  Light Praline Dream, 4-ounce cup
  Light Strawberry Royal, 4-ounce cup
  Low, Light, Luscious Frozen Dairy Dessert, 4-ounce cup

Supermarkets
  Fresh fruit cup or piece of fresh fruit
  Fig Newtons
  Ginger Snaps
  Health Valley fat-free fruit bars or cookies
  Fat-free, sugar-free yogurt

Fat-free, sugar-free yogurt drink
Fat-free, sugar-free fruit muffin
Skim milk
Cut-up raw vegetables
Clear, vegetable-based soup
Applesauce fruit snack
Laughing Cow low-fat cheese wedges
Whole-grain crackers

Food Machines
Peanuts

The Detailed Plans for Eating Out

All diets require more concentration for people who eat out frequently and the G-Index Diet is no exception. The following meal plan assumes the worst possible schedule—that you eat only breakfast at home. Other times, you are eating in restaurants, hotels, in the office, or picking up simple foods in a supermarket. Even then, the G-Index Diet can work for you.

However, eating out does present a question: how big is an ounce of cheese or three ounces of chicken breast? In the ideal world you would weigh your foods before you eat them. In the real world it's nice to have some rough and ready rules to help you pick out serving size.

One ounce of cheese is a chunk about 2″ by 2″ by 1″ high. Prepackaged, presliced ham, roast beef, turkey, or chicken usually has about one ounce per slice. (You can double check by dividing the total number of slices in the package by its total ounces.) Three ounces of chicken breast, veal, beef, or fish is about the same size as a woman's palm. Remember, portion sizes for meats are as they appear cooked. Estimate 25 percent shrinkage from raw to cooked, e.g., from four ounces raw to three ounces cooked.

DAY 1

Meal	Food Item	Location	1,200 Cal	1,500 Cal	1,800 Cal
Breakfast	Extra Fiber All-Bran Cereal	Home, diner, or hotel	⅔ cup	1⅓ cup	1⅓ cup
	blueberries or		¾ cup	1½ cups	1½ cups
	banana		½	1	1
	apple juice or orange juice		—	—	4 oz
	skim milk or nonfat sugar-free fruited yogurt		8 oz	8 oz	8 oz
	decaf coffee or tea		as desired	as desired	as desired
	light nondairy creamer		1 oz	1 oz	1 oz
	or skim milk		2 oz	2 oz	2 oz
Lunch	Wendy's Regular Chili	Wendy's Restaurant	1 serving (9 oz)	1 serving (9 oz)	1 serving (9 oz)
	tossed green salad with low-calorie dressing		3 cups	3 cups	3 cups
			2 tbs	2 tbs	3 tbs

Meal	Food Item	Location	1,200 Cal	1,500 Cal	1,800 Cal
	dried apple chunks (from home)		¾ oz	¾ oz	¾ oz
	or Weight Watchers Fruit Snack (from home)		1 packet	1 packet	1 packet
	water or decaf diet beverage		as desired	as desired	as desired
Snack	Ry Krisp crackers	Home or work	2	2	2
	low-sodium tomato juice or V-8		6 oz	12 oz	12 oz
	water or decaf diet beverage		as desired	as desired	as desired
Dinner	Domino's 16-inch Cheese Pizza	Home delivery	2 slices	2 slices	3 slices
	with onion, mushroom, or pepper topping (optional)		as desired	as desired	as desired
	water or decaf diet beverage		as desired	as desired	as desired

Meal	Food Item	Location	1,200 Cal	1,500 Cal	1,800 Cal
Snack	pear or apple	Diner, hotel, or home	1 large	1 large	1 large
	Swiss cheese		1 oz	2 oz	2 oz
	skim milk or nonfat sugar-free fruited yogurt		—	4 oz	8 oz
	water or decaf diet beverage		as desired	as desired	as desired

DAY 2

Meal	Food Item	Location	1,200 Cal	1,500 Cal	1,800 Cal
Breakfast	whole-grain bread	Diner, hotel, or home	1 slice	1 slice	1 slice
	cottage cheese, 4% milk fat		¼ cup	½ cup	¾ cup
	or diet cheese		1 oz	2 oz	3 oz
	cantaloupe		1 cup	1 cup	2 cups
	or unsweetened applesauce		½ cup	½ cup	1 cup

Meal	Food Item	Location	1,200 Cal	1,500 Cal	1,800 Cal
	skim milk or nonfat sugar-free fruited yogurt		4 oz	4 oz	8 oz
	decaf coffee or tea		as desired	as desired	as desired
	light nondairy creamer		1 oz	1 oz	1 oz
	or skim milk		2 oz	2 oz	2 oz
Lunch	Taco Bell Tostada	Taco Bell restaurant	1	2	2
	apple juice		4 oz	4 oz	8 oz
	or dried apple chunks		¾ oz	¾ oz	1½ oz
	water or decaf diet beverage		as desired	as desired	as desired
Snack	nectarine	Home or work	1 medium	1 medium	1 medium
	or tangerines		3 medium	3 medium	3 medium
	water or decaf diet beverage		as desired	as desired	as desired

Meal	Food Item	Location	1,200 Cal	1,500 Cal	1,800 Cal
Dinner	Chinese take-out: stir-fried chicken	Chinese restaurant	3 oz	3 oz	3 oz
	steamed rice		⅔ cup	⅔ cup	1 cup
	mixed steamed Oriental vegetables		2 cups	3 cups	3 cups
	tossed green salad with vinegar or lemon juice (no oil)		as desired	as desired	as desired
	fresh fruit cup		¾ cup	¾ cup	¾ cup
	water or decaf diet beverage		as desired	as desired	as desired
Snack	skim milk or nonfat sugar-free fruited yogurt	Diner, hotel, or home	8 oz	8 oz	8 oz
	cantaloupe or fresh fruit cup		—	—	1 cup
			—	—	¾ cup

Meal	Food Item	Location	1,200 Cal	1,500 Cal	1,800 Cal
	water or decaf diet beverage		as desired	as desired	as desired

DAY 3

Meal	Food Item	Location	1,200 Cal	1,500 Cal	1,800 Cal
Breakfast	whole-grain bread	Diner, hotel, or home	1 slice	1 slice	2 slices
	sugar-free peanut butter		1 tbs	1 tbs	2 tbs
	blueberries		¾ cup	¾ cup	¾ cup
	or apple		1 small	1 small	1 small
	nonfat sugar-free fruited yogurt		8 oz	8 oz	8 oz
	decaf coffee or tea		as desired	as desired	as desired
	light nondairy creamer		1 oz	1 oz	1 oz
	or skim milk		2 oz	2 oz	2 oz
Lunch	Salad bar: salad greens	Cafeteria, Supermarket, fast-food restaurant, or hotel	3 cups	3 cups	3 cups

Meal	Food Item	Location	1,200 Cal	1,500 Cal	1,800 Cal
	green beans, beets		½ cup	½ cup	½ cup
	broccoli, cauliflower, peppers, tomatoes, onions		2 cups	2 cups	3 cups
	garbanzo beans (chickpeas)		⅓ cup	⅔ cup	⅔ cup
	cottage cheese or flaked tuna		¼ cup	½ cup	½ cup
	reduced-calorie dressing		2 tbs	3 tbs	3 tbs
	Ry Krisp crackers		4	4	4
	cantaloupe or citrus sections		1 cup	1 cup	1 cup
			¾ cup	¾ cup	¾ cup
	water or decaf diet beverage		as desired	as desired	as desired
Snack	apricots or Weight Watchers Fruit Snack	Work or home	4 small	4 large	4 large
			1 packet	2 packets	2 packets
	water or decaf diet beverage		as desired	as desired	as desired

Meal	Food Item	Location	1,200 Cal	1,500 Cal	1,800 Cal
Dinner	Burger King Chicken Tenders	Burger King	6 pieces	6 pieces	6 pieces
	salad greens		3 cups	3 cups	3 cups
	broccoli, cauliflower, peppers, tomatoes, onions		3 cups	3 cups	3 cups
	reduced-calorie dressing		2 tbs	3 tbs	3 tbs
	water or decaf diet beverage		as desired	as desired	as desired
Snack	TCBY (fat-free, sugar-free)	TCBY, diner, hotel, or home	4 oz	4 oz	4 oz
	skim milk		—	4 oz	8 oz
	cherries		12	12	24
	or pear		1 small	1 small	1 large
	water or decaf diet beverage		as desired	as desired	as desired

DAY 4

Meal	Food Item	Location	1,200 Cal	1,500 Cal	1,800 Cal
Breakfast	Carnation Instant Breakfast (diet) with	Home	1 pkg	1 pkg	1 pkg
	skim milk		8 oz	8 oz	8 oz
	Teddy Grahams or Finn Crisp crackers		4	4	4
	with fruit butter or sugar-free jelly		1	1	1
			1 tsp	1 tsp	1 tsp
	pear or apple		1 small	1 small	1 large
	decaf coffee or tea		as desired	as desired	as desired
	light nondairy creamer or skim milk		1 oz	1 oz	1 oz
			2 oz	2 oz	2 oz
Lunch	Salad Bar: salad greens	Cafeteria, super-market, fast-food restaurant or hotel	3 cups	3 cups	3 cups

Meal	Food Item	Location	1,200 Cal	1,500 Cal	1,800 Cal
	green beans, beets		½ cup	1 cup	1 cup
	broccoli, cauliflower, peppers, tomatoes, onions		2 cups	2 cups	3 cups
	garbanzo beans (chickpeas)		⅓ cup	⅔ cup	1 cup
	sunflower seeds		—	—	1 tbs
	turkey or boiled ham		1 oz	2 oz	3 oz
	reduced-calorie dressing		2 tbs	2 tbs	4 tbs
	applesauce		½ cup	½ cup	½ cup
	nonfat sugar-free fruited yogurt		—	8 oz	8 oz
	water or decaf diet beverage		as desired	as desired	as desired
Snack	apricots	Home or work	4 medium	4 medium	4 medium
	or orange		1 small	1 small	1 small
	water or decaf diet beverage		as desired	as desired	as desired

Meal	Food Item	Location	1,200 Cal	1,500 Cal	1,800 Cal
Dinner	Kentucky Fried Original Recipe	KFC restaurant or home			
	Breast		2½ oz	2½ oz	2½ oz
	corn-on-the-cob		1 small ear	1 small ear	1 small ear
	water or decaf diet beverage		as desired	as desired	as desired
Snack	whole-grain bread	Diner, hotel, or home	1 slice	1 slice	1 slice
	diet cheese		1 oz	1 oz	1 oz
	pear or orange		—	1 small	1 small
	skim milk or nonfat sugar-free fruited yogurt		4 oz	4 oz	8 oz
	water or decaf diet beverage		as desired	as desired	as desired

DAY 5

Meal	Food Item	Location	1,200 Cal	1,500 Cal	1,800 Cal
Breakfast	Carnation Instant Breakfast (diet) with skim milk	Home	1 pkg	1 pkg	1 pkg
			8 oz	8 oz	8 oz
	Teddy Grahams or Finn Crisp crackers with fruit butter or sugar-free jelly		4	4	8
			1	1	5
			1 tsp	1 tsp	4 tsp
	fresh berries or		¼ cup	1½ cups	1½ cups
	orange		1 small	1 large	1 large
	decaf coffee or tea		as desired	as desired	as desired
	light nondairy creamer or skim milk		1 oz	1 oz	1 oz
			2 oz	2 oz	2 oz
Lunch	Salad bar: salad greens	Cafeteria, fast-food restaurant, hotel, or home	3 cups	3 cups	3 cups

Meal	Food Item	Location	1,200 Cal	1,500 Cal	1,800 Cal
	green beans & beets		½ cup	1 cup	1 cup
	broccoli, cauliflower, peppers, tomatoes, onions		1 cup	2 cups	2 cups
	garbanzo beans (chickpeas)		⅓ cup	⅔ cup	⅔ cup
	sea legs or flaked tuna		½ cup	¾ cup	¾ cup
	reduced-calorie dressing		4 tbs	6 tbs	6 tbs
	Ry Krisp		4	4	4
	fresh fruit cup or citrus sections		¾ cup	¾ cup	¾ cup
	water or decaf diet beverage		as desired	as desired	as desired
Snack	dried apple chunks	work or home	¾ oz	¾ oz	1½ oz
	or grapes		15 small	15 small	30 small
	water or decaf diet beverage		as desired	as desired	as desired
Dinner	meat lasagna	Italian restaurant, or hotel	8 oz	8 oz	12 oz

Meal	Food Item	Location	1,200 Cal	1,500 Cal	1,800 Cal
	steamed zucchini or grilled eggplant (no oil)		1 cup	1 cup	1 cup
	tossed green salad with vinegar or lemon juice (no oil)		as desired	as desired	as desired
	fresh berries or seasonal fruit cup		¾ cup	¾ cup	¾ cup
	water or decaf diet beverage		as desired	as desired	as desired
Snack	sugar-free gelatin	Diner, hotel, or home	1 cup	1 cup	1 cup
	light whipped topping (optional)		2 tbs	2 tbs	2 tbs
	skim milk		4 oz	4 oz	8 oz
	water or decaf diet beverage		as desired	as desired	as desired

DAY 6

Meal	Food Item	Location	1,200 Cal	1,500 Cal	1,800 Cal
Breakfast	Extra Fiber All-Bran cereal	Diner, hotel, or home	⅓ cup	⅔ cup	⅔ cup
	strawberries		1¼ cups	2½ cups	2½ cups
	or banana		½	1	1
	skim milk or nonfat sugar-free fruited yogurt		8 oz	8 oz	8 oz
	decaf coffee or tea		as desired	as desired	as desired
	light nondairy creamer		1 oz	1 oz	1 oz
	or skim milk		2 oz	2 oz	2 oz
Lunch	pizza with vegetarian topping	Pizzeria	2 slices	2 slices	2 slices
	water or decaf diet beverage		as desired	as desired	as desired
Snack	kiwi or orange	work or home	1	1	1
	water or decaf diet beverage		as desired	as desired	as desired

Meal	Food Item	Location	1,200 Cal	1,500 Cal	1,800 Cal
	old-fashioned vegetable soup		1 cup	1 cup	1 cup
Dinner	sirloin steak	Diner, steak house, or hotel	3 oz	4 oz	5 oz
	baked potato		1 medium	1 medium	1 large
	with margarine		1 pat	2 pats	3 pats
	tossed green salad		3 cups	3 cups	3 cups
	with reduced-calorie dressing		2 tbs	2 tbs	2 tbs
	steamed green beans		1 cup	2 cups	2 cups
	fresh fruit cup		¼ cup	¼ cup	¼ cup
	water or decaf diet beverage		as desired	as desired	as desired
Snack	skim milk or nonfat sugar-free fruited yogurt	Diner or home	4 oz	4 oz	8 oz

Meal	Food Item	Location	1,200 Cal	1,500 Cal	1,800 Cal
	fresh berries or seasonal fruit cup		¾ cup	¾ cup	1½ cups
	water or decaf diet beverage		as desired	as desired	as desired

DAY 7

Meal	Food Item	Location	1,200 Cal	1,500 Cal	1,800 Cal
Breakfast	whole-grain bread	Diner, hotel, or home	1 slice	1 slice	1 slice
	scrambled or fried egg (egg substitute optional)		1	1	1
	orange juice or		4 oz	8 oz	8 oz
	grapefruit		½	1	1
	margarine		—	1 pat	1 pat
	skim milk or nonfat sugar-free fruited yogurt		4 oz	8 oz	8 oz

Meal	Food Item	Location	1,200 Cal	1,500 Cal	1,800 Cal
	decaf coffee or tea		as desired	as desired	as desired
	light nondairy creamer		1 oz	1 oz	1 oz
	or skim milk		2 oz	2 oz	2 oz
Lunch	Ry Krisp crackers	Diner, hotel, or home	4	6	8
	part-skim mozzarella cheese		2 oz	3 oz	4 oz
	or part-skim ricotta cheese		½ cup	¾ cup	1 cup
	grilled pepper strips (no oil)		1 cup	1 cup	2 cups
	or tomato juice or V-8		6 oz	6 oz	12 oz
	banana		1 large	1 large	1 large
	or fresh berries		1½ cups	1½ cups	1½ cups
	water or decaf diet beverage		as desired	as desired	as desired
Snack	skim milk or nonfat sugar-free fruited yogurt	Diner, hotel, or home	8 oz	8 oz	8 oz

Meal	Food Item	Location	1,200 Cal	1,500 Cal	1,800 Cal
	water or decaf diet beverage		as desired	as desired	as desired
Dinner	beef enchilada	Mexican restaurant	1	1	2
	chili & beans		½ cup	½ cup	½ cup
	tossed green salad with vinegar or lemon juice (no oil)		as desired	as desired	as desired
	steamed zucchini in hot tomato sauce		1 cup	1½ cups	1½ cups
	water or decaf diet beverage		as desired	as desired	as desired
Snack	sugar-free gelatin	Diner, hotel, or home	1 cup	1 cup	1 cup
	light whipped topping (optional)		2 tbs	2 tbs	2 tbs
	strawberries or		1¼ cups	1¼ cups	2½ cups
	orange		1 small	1 small	1 large
	water or decaf diet beverage		as desired	as desired	as desired

DAY 8

Meal	Food Item	Location	1,200 Cal	1,500 Cal	1,800 Cal
Breakfast	Carnation Instant Breakfast (diet) with skim	Home	1 pkg	1 pkg	1 pkg
	milk		8 oz	8 oz	8 oz
	Teddy Grahams or Finn Crisp		4	4	4
	crackers with fruit butter or sugar-free		4	4	4
	jelly		4 tsp	4 tsp	4 tsp
	cantaloupe		1 cup	2 cups	2 cups
	or pear		1 small	1 large	1 large
	decaf coffee or tea		as desired	as desired	as desired
	light nondairy creamer		1 oz	1 oz	1 oz
	or skim milk		2 oz	2 oz	2 oz
Lunch	mushroom crepes	Continental restaurant or hotel	2–3 oz	2–3 oz	2–3 oz
	tossed green salad		3 cups	3 cups	3 cups

Meal	Food Item	Location	1,200 Cal	1,500 Cal	1,800 Cal
	with vinegar or lemon juice (no oil)		as desired	as desired	as desired
	stir-fried garden vegetables		—	—	2 cups
	stewed peaches with mint raspberry sauce		½ cup	½ cup	½ cup
	or cantaloupe		1½ cups	1½ cups	1½ cups
	water or decaf diet beverage		as desired	as desired	as desired
Snack	nectarine or orange	work or home	1 small	1 small	1 large
	water or decaf diet beverage		as desired	as desired	as desired
Dinner	Manhattan clam or tomato corn chowder	Diner, hotel, or American-style restaurant	1 cup	1 cup	2 cups (bowl)
	or vegetable or lentil soup		1½ cups	1½ cups	3 cups

Meal	Food Item	Location	1,200 Cal	1,500 Cal	1,800 Cal
	broiled swordfish with lemon		5 oz	6 oz	7 oz
	boiled parslied potato		1 small	1 medium	1 medium
	stewed tomatoes or steamed asparagus with margarine		1 cup	1½ cups	1½ cups
			1 pat	2 pats	2 pats
	fresh berries or seasonal fruit cup		¼ cup	¼ cup	¼ cup
	water or decaf diet beverage		as desired	as desired	as desired
Snack	skim milk or nonfat sugar-free fruited yogurt	Diner, hotel, or home	4 oz	8 oz	8 oz
	water or decaf diet beverage		as desired	as desired	as desired

DAY 9

Meal	Food Item	Location	1,200 Cal	1,500 Cal	1,800 Cal
Breakfast	old-fashioned oatmeal	Diner, hotel, or home	½ cup	½ cup	1 cup
	orange juice or unsweetened applesauce		4 oz	4 oz	4 oz
			½ cup	½ cup	½ cup
	skim milk or nonfat sugar-free fruited yogurt		8 oz	8 oz	8 oz
	decaf coffee or tea		as desired	as desired	as desired
	light nondairy creamer or skim milk		1 oz	1 oz	1 oz
			2 oz	2 oz	2 oz
Lunch	pizza primavera	Pizzeria	2 slices	2 slices	2 slices
	nonfat sugar-free frozen yogurt		4 oz	4 oz	4 oz
	water or decaf diet beverage		as desired	as desired	as desired
Snack	pear	work or home	1 small	1 large	1 large

Meal	Food Item	Location	1,200 Cal	1,500 Cal	1,800 Cal
	or Real Fruit Bar		1 bar	2 bars	2 bars
	dry roasted almonds		—	6	12
	water or decaf diet beverage		as desired	as desired	as desired
Dinner	wonton soup	Chinese restaurant	1 cup	1 cup	1 cup
	shrimp or chicken lo mein		1 cup	1 cup	2 cups
	steamed rice		⅓ cup	⅔ cup	⅔ cup
	fresh fruit cup		¾ cup	¾ cup	¾ cup
	water or decaf diet beverage		as desired	as desired	as desired
`nack	cheddar or Swiss cheese	Diner, hotel, or home	1½ oz	1½ oz	1½ oz
	peach or apple		1 small	1 small	1 large
	skim milk or nonfat sugar-free fruited yogurt		—	8 oz	8 oz
	water or decaf diet beverage		as desired	as desired	as desired

DAY 10

Meal	Food Item	Location	1,200 Cal	1,500 Cal	1,800 Cal
Breakfast	whole-grain bread	Diner, hotel, or home	1 slice	1 slice	2 slices
	light cream cheese		1 oz	1 oz	1 oz
	fresh berries		¾ cup	¾ cup	¾ cup
	or pear		1 small	1 small	1 small
	skim milk or nonfat sugar-free fruited yogurt		8 oz	8 oz	8 oz
	decaf coffee or tea		as desired	as desired	as desired
	light nondairy creamer		1 oz	1 oz	1 oz
	or skim milk		2 oz	2 oz	2 oz
Lunch	chicken fajita with sautéed onions, peppers,	Contemporary-style restaurant	1	1	1
	salsa		½ cup	½ cup	½ cup
	tossed green salad		3 cups	3 cups	3 cups

Meal	Food Item	Location	1,200 Cal	1,500 Cal	1,800 Cal
	with vinegar or lemon juice (no oil)		as desired	as desired	as desired
	fresh berries or seasonal fruit cup		¾ cup	¾ cup	1½ cups
	water or decaf diet beverage		as desired	as desired	as desired
Snack	Real Fruit Bar or apple	work or home	1 bar 1 small	1 bar 1 small	1 bar 1 small
	Teddy Grahams or Finn Crisp crackers with fruit butter or sugar-free jelly		— —	— —	15 4 4 tsp
	water or decaf diet beverage		as desired	as desired	as desired

Meal	Food Item	Location	1,200 Cal	1,500 Cal	1,800 Cal
Dinner	broiled cod or haddock steak	Fish, Continental, or American-style restaurant	5½ oz	7½ oz	7½ oz
	steamed rice		⅓ cup	⅔ cup	⅔ cup
	stir-fried vegetables		2 cups	3 cups	3 cups
	tossed green salad with vinegar or lemon juice (no oil)		3 cups	3 cups	3 cups
	nonfat sugar-free frozen yogurt		as desired	as desired	as desired
	water or decaf diet beverage		⅓ cup	⅓ cup	⅓ cup
			as desired	as desired	as desired
Snack	graham cracker squares	Diner, hotel, or home	3	3	3
	part-skim mozzarella cheese or part-skim ricotta cheese		—	1 oz	1 oz
			—	¼ cup	¼ cup

Meal	Food Item	Location	1,200 Cal	1,500 Cal	1,800 Cal
	stewed fruit or unsweetened applesauce		½ cup	1 cup	1 cup
	skim milk or nonfat sugar-free fruited yogurt		—	—	8 oz
	water or decaf diet beverage		as desired	as desired	as desired

DAY 11

Meal	Food Item	Location	1,200 Cal	1,500 Cal	1,800 Cal
Breakfast	whole-grain bread	Diner, hotel, or home	1 slice	1 slice	1 slice
	plain omelet		1 egg	1 egg	1 egg
	grapefruit or orange		½	1	1
	juice		4 oz	8 oz	8 oz
	skim milk or nonfat sugar-free fruited yogurt		4 oz	4 oz	4 oz

Meal	Food Item	Location	1,200 Cal	1,500 Cal	1,800 Cal
	decaf coffee or tea		as desired	as desired	as desired
	light nondairy creamer		1 oz	1 oz	1 oz
	or skim milk		2 oz	2 oz	2 oz
Lunch	roast turkey breast	Diner, hotel, or American-style restaurant	3 oz	4 oz	4 oz
	peas		1 cup	1 cup	1 cup
	sautéed cauliflower & scallions		½ cup	1 cup	1 cup
	or braised zucchini or leeks		½ cup	1 cup	1 cup
	seasonal fruit compote		¾ cup	¾ cup	¾ cup
	water or decaf diet beverage		as desired	as desired	as desired
Snack	graham cracker squares	work or home	—	—	3
	skim milk or nonfat sugar-free fruited yogurt		8 oz	8 oz	8 oz

Meal	Food Item	Location	1,200 Cal	1,500 Cal	1,800 Cal
	water or decaf diet beverage		as desired	as desired	as desired
Dinner	cheese ravioli (1 oz size) with tomato	Italian restaurant	8 (1 oz each)	8 (1 oz each)	12 (1 oz each)
	sauce		¼ cup	¼ cup	½ cup
	tossed green salad with vinegar or lemon juice (no oil)		3 cups	3 cups	3 cups
	steamed broccoli or eggplant with garlic &		as desired	as desired	as desired
	parsley		1 cup	1 cup	1 cup
	fresh fruit cup		—	—	¾ cup
	meringue (optional)		1 large	1 large	1 large
	water or decaf diet beverage		as desired	as desired	as desired
Snack	apple or orange	Diner, hotel, or home	1 small	1 large	1 large

Meal	Food Item	Location	1,200 Cal	1,500 Cal	1,800 Cal
	skim milk or nonfat sugar-free fruited yogurt		—	4 oz	4 oz
	water or decaf diet beverage		as desired	as desired	as desired

DAY 12

Meal	Food Item	Location	1,200 Cal	1,500 Cal	1,800 Cal
Breakfast	Carnation Instant Breakfast (diet) with	Home	1 pkg	1 pkg	1 pkg
	skim milk		8 oz	8 oz	8 oz
	Teddy Grahams or Finn Crisp		4	4	19
	crackers with fruit butter or sugar-free jelly		1	1	5
			1 tsp	1 tsp	1 tbsp
	peach or apple		1 small	1 large	1 large

Meal	Food Item	Location	1,200 Cal	1,500 Cal	1,800 Cal
	decaf coffee or tea		as desired	as desired	as desired
	light nondairy creamer		1 oz	1 oz	1 oz
	or skim milk		2 oz	2 oz	2 oz
Lunch	chili con carne & beans (no toppings)	Diner or Mexican restaurant	7 oz	7 oz	7 oz
	tossed green salad with assorted raw vegetables		3 cups	3 cups	3 cups
	with reduced-calorie		1 cup	1 cup	1 cup
	dressing		2 tbs	2 tbs	4 tbs
	apple juice		4 oz	8 oz	12 oz
	water or decaf diet beverage		as desired	as desired	as desired
Snack	Teddy Grahams or Finn Crisp	work or home	8	8	8
	crackers		2	2	2

Meal	Food Item	Location	1,200 Cal	1,500 Cal	1,800 Cal
	with fruit butter or sugar-free jelly		2 tsp	2 tsp	2 tsp
	skim milk or nonfat sugar-free fruited jelly		4 oz	8 oz	8 oz
	water or decaf diet beverage		as desired	as desired	as desired
Dinner	breast of chicken, poached	Hotel or continental restaurant			
	in wine		3 oz	4 ½ oz	5 ½ oz
	steamed rice		⅔ cup	1 cup	1 cup
	sliced tomatoes		1 cup	1 cup	1 cup
	with vinaigrette dressing		1 tbs	1 tbs	1 tbs
	fresh citrus sections or seasonal fruit compote		¾ cup	¾ cup	¾ cup
	water or decaf diet beverage		as desired	as desired	as desired

Meal	Food Item	Location	1,200 Cal	1,500 Cal	1,800 Cal
Snack	mixed berries or seasonal fruit cup	Diner, hotel, or home	¾ cup	¾ cup	¾ cup
	light whipped topping (optional)		2 tbs	2 tbs	2 tbs
	water or decaf diet beverage		as desired	as desired	as desired

DAY 13

Meal	Food Item	Location	1,200 Cal	1,500 Cal	1,800 Cal
Breakfast	bran muffin	Diner, hotel, or home	1 small (2 oz)	1 med. (4 oz)	1 med. (4 oz)
	sugar-free peanut butter		1 tbs	1 tbs	1 tbs
	grapefruit		½	½	½
	or orange juice		4 oz	4 oz	4 oz
	skim milk or nonfat sugar-free fruited yogurt		4 oz	4 oz	8 oz

Meal	Food Item	Location	1,200 Cal	1,500 Cal	1,800 Cal
	decaf coffee or tea		as desired	as desired	as desired
	light nondairy creamer		1 oz	1 oz	1 oz
	or skim milk		2 oz	2 oz	2 oz
Lunch	beef vegetable & barley soup	Diner, hotel, or American-style restaurant	2 cups (bowl)	2 cups (bowl)	2 cups (bowl)
	or chicken with rice		1½ cups	1½ cups	1½ cups
	whole-grain bread		1 slice	1 slice	2 slices
	boiled ham or turkey breast		1 oz	1 oz	2 oz
	mustard (optional)		1 tsp	1 tsp	1 tsp
	celery & cucumber sticks		1 cup	1 cup	2 cups
	or tossed green salad with assorted raw vegetables		3 cups	3 cups	3 cups
			1 cup	1 cup	2 cups

Meal	Food Item	Location	1,200 Cal	1,500 Cal	1,800 Cal
	with vinegar or lemon juice (no oil)		as desired	as desired	as desired
	fresh fruit cup		¾ cup	¾ cup	¾ cup
	water or decaf diet beverage		as desired	as desired	as desired
Snack	nectarine or apple	work or home	1 small	1 large	1 large
	water or decaf diet beverage		as desired	as desired	as desired
Dinner	broiled turkey tenders with lemon	steak house or American-style restaurant	3 oz	4 oz	4 oz
	boiled parslied potato		1 medium	1 medium	1 medium
	grilled onions		½ cup	1 cup	1 cup
	steamed green beans or spinach		½ cup	1 cup	1 cup

Meal	Food Item	Location	1,200 Cal	1,500 Cal	1,800 Cal
	with margarine		—	—	1 pat
	fresh berries or fresh fruit cup		¾ cup	¾ cup	1½ cups
	water or decaf diet beverage		as desired	as desired	as desired
Snack	skim milk or nonfat sugar-free fruited yogurt	Diner, hotel, or home	8 oz	8 oz	8 oz
	or nonfat, sugar-free frozen fruit yogurt		4 oz	4 oz	4 oz
	water or decaf diet beverage		as desired	as desired	as desired

DAY 14

Meal	Food Item	Location	1,200 Cal	1,500 Cal	1,800 Cal
Breakfast	old-fashioned oatmeal	Diner, hotel, or home	½ cup	½ cup	1 cup

Meal	Food Item	Location	1,200 Cal	1,500 Cal	1,800 Cal
	whole-grain bread		1 slice	1 slice	1 slice
	egg, soft-boiled or poached		1	1	1
	blueberries or		¾ cup	¾ cup	¾ cup
	orange juice		4 oz	4 oz	4 oz
	skim milk or nonfat sugar-free fruited yogurt		4 oz	8 oz	8 oz
	decaf coffee or tea		as desired	as desired	as desired
	light nondairy creamer		1 oz	1 oz	1 oz
	or skim milk		2 oz	2 oz	2 oz
Lunch	lentil soup, clam chowder, or minestrone	Diner, hotel, or home	8 oz	8 oz	8 oz
	Ry Krisp crackers		—	4	4
	part-skim mozzarella cheese		—	¼ cup	½ cup

Meal	Food Item	Location	1,200 Cal	1,500 Cal	1,800 Cal
	or part-skim ricotta cheese		—	¼ cup	½ cup
	tossed green salad with assorted raw vegetables		3 cups	3 cups	3 cups
	with vinegar or lemon juice (no oil)		2 cups	2 cups	2 cups
			as desired	as desired	as desired
	apple or orange		1 small	1 large	1 large
	water or decaf diet beverage		as desired	as desired	as desired
Snack	skim milk or nonfat sugar-free fruited yogurt	work or home	4 oz	4 oz	4 oz
	water or decaf diet beverage		as desired	as desired	as desired
Dinner	butterfly pasta	Hotel or Italian restaurant	1 cup	1 cup	1 cup

Meal	Food Item	Location	1,200 Cal	1,500 Cal	1,800 Cal
	with salmon sauce		½ cup	½ cup	½ cup
	or sugar-free tomato sauce		½ cup	½ cup	½ cup
	with meatballs (1 oz size)		3	3	3
	spinach salad (no bacon bits)		3 cups	3 cups	3 cups
	with vinaigrette dressing		1 tbs	1 tbs	1 tbs
	grilled eggplant or zucchini (no oil)		½ cup	1 cup	1½ cups
	lemon sorbet		½ cup	½ cup	½ cup
	water or decaf diet beverage		as desired	as desired	as desired
Snack	fresh fruit cup	Diner, hotel, or home	¾ cup	¾ cup	1½ cups
	skim milk or nonfat sugar-free fruited				

Meal	Food Item	Location	1,200 Cal	1,500 Cal	1,800 Cal
	water or decaf diet beverage		as desired	as desired	as desired

CHAPTER NINE

Quick Takes: Simple Foods and Snacks

Snacks are a dirty word with many dieters. But as you begin to develop a more flexible approach to the G-Index Diet, you'll find that snacks are an extremely important mini-meal that can carry you over the natural blood-sugar dips that occur between meals.

In this chapter, you'll learn more about the rationale behind the snacks you've been using on the fixed G-Index menus. You'll also learn how to wield your "snack power" more freely as you put together your own diet. But first, here's an overview of the snack possibilities you'll be encountering.

A GUIDE TO G-INDEX SNACKS

There are four calorie levels of snack listings in the latter part of this chapter:

1. Very low calorie (fewer than 20 calories) or no-calorie snacks
2. 60-calorie snacks
3. 120-calorie snacks
4. 200-calorie snacks

If you like, begin to design your own meal plan right now by substituting some of these snacks for the ones in the fixed menus. People on the 1,200-calorie G-Index diet should select one snack for each of their two daily snack times from the 60-calorie snack list. People on the 1,500-calorie diet should also pick one snack at each snack time from the 60-calorie list.

People on the 1,800-calorie diet can divide their snacks this way: eat 120 calories for the afternoon snack and 120 calories for the evening snack; or, take in 200 calories at one of the snack times and 60 calories at the other.

People who are relatively large, active, or muscular may find that they can eat more food at snack time and still maintain their weight. If you are in this category, feel free to add an extra item or two from the snack lists. But be sure to monitor your weight to see that you're not taking in so much extra food that you're starting to regain lost weight!

You should *not* take in all your snack calories at one snack time and then skip the other snack. It's important to keep feeding your system throughout the day to achieve maximum burning of calories.

When Should You Eat a Snack?

The common times for snacks are mid-morning, afternoon, and late evening. I scheduled only two snacks per day in the fixed menus, however, because I've found that eating a solid, low GI breakfast can help most people stay satisfied until lunchtime. I suggest that you follow this plan as you design your own G-Index program.

Now, here are some further thoughts on snack times.

- *Morning Snack—A Marginal Proposition*. As I've said, for most people a low G-Index breakfast eliminates the need for a late-morning snack. Consequently, you should be able to skip this mini-meal.

  But others find they do need a mid-morning snack, perhaps because they have an exceptionally high metabolism or their morning activity causes them to burn up an inordinate number of calories. Or the office may "require" a morning coffee break.

In such situations, choose a *very* low-calorie, low-G-Index food. Pick them from the no-calorie, very-low-calorie, or 60-calorie listings later in this chapter. The snack might consist of a fruit, a slice of pumpernickel bread, or a half-cup of nonfat, low G-Index yogurt.

Never choose a high G-Index food as your main snack. If you do, you'll regret it because your appetite will probably go out of control.

- *Afternoon Snack.* Many, if not most, people are better off with a late-afternoon snack. For one thing, eating at this time helps you handle the mid-afternoon blood sugar dip. Also, an afternoon snack helps keep your blood sugar levels steady so you won't become ravenous by the time you eat dinner at 6:00 or 7:00 P.M., or later.

  Also, the low G-Index, late-afternoon snack reduces appetite and improves the likelihood that you'll make good food selection choices at dinner. For example, you'll be less tempted to gorge on bread or some other high GI item before you get around to the main part of the meal.

  Did you ever wonder why restaurants serve bread before you order? They're certainly not trying to fill you up so that you eat less! They've found through experience that people who overdose on bread tend to order and eat more.

- *Evening Snack.* This snack, which would typically be eaten before bed, provides a slow, steady flow of nutrition during the night. The result is reduced hunger and appetite the next morning.

  In contrast, a high G-Index snack or meal the night before leads to a craving for more and higher G-Index foods the next morning.

Additional Snack Tactics

It's important to evaluate the snack situation you're confronting and then choose the *lowest calorie snack that will satisfy your needs.* You don't want to attack a fly with a piece of artillery! Similarly, you don't want to overeat at snack time when you can satisfy yourself just as well with less food.

Snack Tactic 1. *Identify situations that call for very-low or no-calorie food.* You may not be hungry at all, but you need a chance to chew, taste, or pass the time away. Perhaps your work or social situation coerces you to eat. For example, you may be served something to nibble on just before a dinner party. In these situations, it's best not to waste your allotted calories for the day when you can get by with few or no calories. A club soda with lime may satisfy you completely— so why eat a high-fat hors d'oeuvre?

To meet the needs of this kind of snacking, I've provided a list of low GI snacks that contain 20 calories or less. You may eat up to two or three servings a day of the foods listed that have no specific serving size. Eat as much as you want of all the others. Try to spread them out during the day.

Snack Tactic 2. *Identify situations that call for regular nutritional snacks.* If you really are hungry between meals or you're scheduled for a regular snack, you'll want an instant hunger stopper that's tasty, convenient, and low on the Glycemic Index. Depending on how hungry you are, how long you'll have to wait until the next meal, and the calorie level of your diet, you should select a snack of 60, 120, or 200 calories from the lists I've included.

Snack Tactic 3. *Identify situations that call for meal substitutes.* Sometimes you may find yourself dashing out of the house without time to prepare a regular meal. Or perhaps you've forgotten to plan your meal. So you decide it would be best to put something together quickly from the cold dishes, raw vegetables, fruits, leftovers, or other items readily available in your kitchen.

In these emergency circumstances, you'll probably find that consuming low GI foods containing 300 to 500 calories will satisfy you. One way to meet this need is to rely on frozen foods, described after the 200-calorie selections later in this chapter.

Another way to construct a satisfying low GI meal substitute is to take two or three items from the 60-, 120-, or 200-calorie snack listings, so that you have a total of up to about 300 to 500 calories. (People eating at the 1,200-calorie level should go for a 300-calorie meal substitute; those on the 1,500-calorie diet, a 400-calorie substitute; and those on the 1,800-calorie diet, a 500-calorie substitute.)

People who occasionally put together snack components as a meal substitute should concentrate on dairy foods and fruits. For example, a person who needs a 500-calorie meal substitute might choose 6 ounces of low-fat cottage cheese, one of our Apples 'n' Oats muffins (page 136), and a piece of low GI fruit such as a pear or grapefruit. This meal substitute provides enough energy to make it to the next snack, and also the nutrients feed into the bloodstream slowly because of the low GI quality of the food.

Always Be Aware of the Dangers!

Snacks in the mid-afternoon are usually *necessary* to help most people make it through the day—even if low GI foods have been consumed at the previous meal. At the same time, snacks are among the most vulnerable times for triggering surges in blood sugar, insulin, and appetite. They may become dangerous in two ways:

- Snack eating can go out of control if the previous meal includes high G-Index foods. The drop in blood sugar will be exaggerated two to four hours after eating, and the result will be severe hunger. It will be difficult or impossible to control your intake of food, as you strive to bring your blood sugar back again to a comfortable level. Under these stressful circumstances, it's easy to make unwise food choices at snack time. People with a hypoglycemic tendency suffer worse from this phenomenon, but *everyone* who eats high GI foods is affected to some extent.
- Eating a high GI snack will trigger appetite *after* the snack, but usually *before* the next meal. In other words,

snacks must be composed of low GI foods if they are to be effective, otherwise, they won't last long enough. They'll cause that sharp upsurge in sugar and insulin, and you will be tempted to consume high GI foods just before or during the next meal to counter the hunger.

How do you avoid these danger zones? The best way is to pre-select your favorite G-Index snacks at the four major calorie levels. Then you'll be ready to turn to one of these instant hunger-stoppers whenever your appetite begins to get out of hand.

The American Dietetics Association defines "free foods" as those containing 20 calories or less. These make excellent snacks without adding enough calories to matter. Their effect on the G-Index and blood sugar metabolism is also not an issue. You may eat 2-3 servings a day of free foods. In most cases—within reason—you do not need to pay attention to portion size.

Please refer to pages 74–76 for the list of "free foods."

Our more weighty snacks are listed below.

Abbreviations: F = high fat (strictly limit portion size);
S = high salt (more than 400 mg/serving).

60-CALORIE G-INDEX SNACKS—INSTANT HUNGER-STOPPERS

Food	Amount
BREAD AND CRACKERS (may add "free food" sugar-free jelly)	
low G-index bread (see list page 54)	1 slice
Ry Krisp, Wasa Crispbread, or whole-grain rye cracker	4 large
Scandinavian Bran Crispbread-type bran crackers	5 crackers

Food	Amount
diet bread (high G-Index)	1 slice
with diet margarine or light	
cream cheese	1–2 teaspoons

(Comment: This combination of high G-Index carbohydrate and a fat has a lower G-index than the carbohydrate alone.)

COOKIES AND MUFFINS

graham crackers	1 double
Fig Newton	1
R. W. Frookie (high-fructose)	
cookie	2
R. W. Frookie Apple Fruitin	
Cookie	1

(See low G-Index muffin, cracker, and snack list, pages 58–60.)

DAIRY FOODS

buttermilk	½ cup
cheese, fat-free—e.g.,	
Weight Watchers	2 ounces
cheese, partly fat-free	1 ounce
cheese, full-fat	1 ounce (F)
cottage cheese, 2% fat	2 ounces
cottage cheese, 1% fat	3 ounces
cottage cheese, nonfat	4 ounces
feta cheese	1 ounce
Fruit Frappe (GI recipe)	½ cup
milk, skim or 1%	
yogurt, no fat, plain	5 ounces
yogurt, no fat, fruited,	
sugar-free	4 ounces

DAIRY, FROZEN

Weight Watchers Chocolate	
Mousse	2 popsicles

Food	Amount
Cream pops—Good Humor Creamsicle	2 popsicles

DAIRY, HOT

Weight Watchers Hot Cocoa Mix (made with water)	1 envelope

EGGS

egg, boiled	1 egg
egg substitute, low-fat type, e.g., Egg Beaters	½ cup
egg white, fried with nonstick spray	4 egg whites

FATTY FOODS (F)

olives	10 small or 5 large (S)

FRUIT

apple, small	1
applesauce, unsweetened	½ cup
apricot, raw	4 medium
apricot, canned	½ cup or 4 halves
blackberries	¾ cup
blueberries	¾ cup
cantaloupe	⅓ melon or 1 cup cubes
cherries, raw	12 large
cherries, canned	½ cup
fruit cocktail, canned	½ cup
grapefruit	½ medium or ¾ cup segments
grapes, small	15 grapes
honeydew melon	⅛ medium or 1 cup cubes
nectarine	1 nectarine
orange	1 orange
peach, raw	1 whole or ¾ cup pieces
peaches, canned	½ cup or 2 halves

Food	Amount
pear, raw	½ large or 1 small
pears, canned	½ cup or 2 halves
plums	2
raspberries	1 cup
strawberries	1¼ cups
tangerine	2

FRUIT JUICE (no sugar added)

apple, cranberry juice cocktail, grape juice, grapefruit, orange juice, or mixed juices	½ cup
spritzer of half fruit juice, half sparkling water	1 cup
frozen fruit juice, homemade or commercial—e.g., Froze Fruit	1 popsicle
fruit bar—e.g., Nature's Choice Real Fruit Bar	1 roll

SOUPS

Campbell's Healthy Request Hearty Chicken Noodle or Hearty Minestrone	6 ounces

VEGETABLES

any vegetable*	2 cups raw or 1 cup cooked

*Vegetables include artichoke, asparagus, green beans, bean sprouts, broccoli, Brussels sprouts, cabbage, cauliflower, eggplant, greens (collard, mustard, turnip), kohlrabi, leeks, mushrooms, okra, onions, snowpeas, peppers, rutabaga, sauerkraut (S), summer squash, tomato, turnips, water chestnuts, and zucchini.

Carrots, the one important high G-Index vegetable, are limited to 1 large per day (35 calories) and must never be eaten alone. Eat carrots with a small fruit or 1 cup vegetables.

Food	Amount
any vegetable juice except carrot juice	1 cup
mixed vegetable juices—V-8	1 cup
cold boiled potato	1 small

120-CALORIE SNACKS—MORE INSTANT HUNGER-STOPPERS

Food	Amount

BREADS AND CRACKERS (May add "free food" sugar-free jelly)

low G-index bread with	1 slice
diet margarine or	1 tablespoon
all-fruit jelly	2 teaspoons
Ry Krisp	6 triple crackers
matzoh 100% stoneground whole wheat—e.g., Goodman's, Manischewitz	1 board
toasted pita with 1 teaspoon diet margarine	1 small
45-calorie diet bread with 55-calories/ounces cheese, melted	1 slice
	1 ounce

COOKIES AND MUFFINS

cookies with fructose sweetener—e.g., Fifty 50 Chocolate Chip Diabetic Cookies or R. W. Frookie	3
Fruit and Fitness Cookies	3
graham crackers	2 double
Fruit-sweetened bars and muffins—e.g., Health Valley Fat-Free Apple-Fruit Bars	1

Food	Amount
Health Valley Fat-Free Apple Spice Muffin	1, 2 ounces
Health Valley Fat-Free Date Delight Cookies	2
Health Valley Fat-Free Granola Bar	1
Muffin-a-Day	1, 3.8 ounces
Nature's Choice Oat Bran Bars	1
Apples 'N' Oats Muffin (GI recipe)	1 muffin

DAIRY FOODS

Food	Amount
buttermilk	1 cup
cottage cheese, regular (4.2% milk fat)	4 ounces
cottage cheese, low-fat (0.3% milk fat)	7 ounces
full-fat cheese	1 ounce (F) (S)
Imitation cheese—e.g., Tofurella milk-free soy product	1.5 ounces
skim or 1% milk	11 ounces
skim milk with sugar-free hot cocoa mix	7 ounces
plain nonfat yogurt	11 ounces
plain nonfat yogurt mixed with sliced ½ small apple, ¼ banana, ½ cup berries, cantaloupe or honeydew melon	8 ounces or ½ cup
fruited yogurt, fat-free, no added sugar	10 ounces
frozen yogurt, nonfat, sugar-free	4–5 ounces
Fruit Frappe (GI recipe)	8 ounces

Food	Amount

FAT FOODS (F)—Portion Sizes Strictly Limited
   (These are best used as part of a snack along with a carbohydrate or protein food.)

almonds	16 whole
anchovies	1.5 ounces
olives	20 small or 10 large
pecans	14 halves
pignolia nuts	1 tablespoon
peanut butter—e.g., on celery	1 tablespoon
peanuts	25 large

FRUIT

See 60-calorie list	double the serving—usually 1 large or 2 small pieces

FRUIT JUICE

See 60-calorie list	1 cup juice as shown or mixed fruit juices
frozen fruit juice, homemade or commercial—e.g., Froze Fruit	one popsicle
fruit salad—e.g., finely chopped ½ small apple, finely chopped ½ orange, sliced ½ grapefruit, 8 grapes, sliced honeydew, sliced ¼ cantaloupe, 1 tablespoon shredded coconut	1½ cups

SOUPS

Health Valley Mushroom Barley	½ 15-ounce can
Health Valley Tomato	½ 15-ounce can
Progresso Lentil	10.5-ounce can (S)

Food	Amount
Progresso Green Split Pea	½ 19-ounce can (S)
Pritikin Vegetable Soup	14¾-ounce can
Rokeach (Kosher) Barley and Mushroom	10¾-ounce can (S)

VEGETARIAN DISHES AND BEANS

Food	Amount
Taste Adventure Lentil Chili	6 ounces
mixed veggies in pita pocket, with low-calorie dressing	1 pocket
potato, boiled, with 2 tablespoons imitation sour cream	1 small
Amy's Mexican Tamale Pie	8 ounces

200-CALORIE SNACKS—LARGER HUNGER-STOPPERS

Food	Amount

BREADS AND CRACKERS

Food	Amount
low G-Index bread	1 slice
with lean meat, poultry, fish,	2 ounces
or low-fat cheese	1–2 ounces
sprouted whole wheat bagel— e.g., Alvarado Street	1

COOKIES AND MUFFINS

Food	Amount
R. W. Frookie	4
Apples 'N' Oats Muffins (GI recipe) plus 1 tablespoon sugar-free jelly	1
Nature's Warehouse Juice-Flavored Pastry Popover	1

Food	Amount
Muffin–A–Day Brand Health Muffins	1

DAIRY FOODS

Food	Amount
full-fat cheese with fruit	1 ounce (F) + 1 fruit
part-skim cheese with fruit	2 ounces + 1 fruit
flavored milk drink—e.g., Carnation Instant Breakfast	1 packet + 1 cup 2% milk
cottage cheese, low-fat plus fruit, cantaloupe, or berries	6 ounces cottage cheese plus 1 fruit or ⅓ cantaloupe or 1 cup berries
plain non-sugar, non-fat yogurt with sliced apple, banana, berries, or melon, sweetened with fructose— mixed or pureed	8 ounces yogurt plus 1 apple, or ½ banana or 1 cup berries or 1 cup melon with 1 or 2 15-calorie packets of fructose
Ultra Slim-Fast, Vanilla (Chocolate has 20 more calories)	12 ounces

FATTY FOODS

Food	Amount
sunflower seeds, unsalted	4 tablespoons

PROTEIN FOODS

Food	Amount
tuna, in water; turkey; light meat chicken	6 ounces
rare roast beef; cured, lean ham	4 ounces
tuna (light), in water, with 1 tablespoon low-calorie mayonnaise, 1 slice 45-calorie low GI bread, lettuce, tomato slice	3 ounces tuna and one slice low GI bread, lettuce and tomato

MEAL SUBSTITUTES

The majority of meals in the 21-day menus can be prepared in thirty minutes or less. Most snacks require no preparation at all. As you read through the menus, make note of which foods you want to keep on hand to "grab" when you are in a hurry.

You should also become familiar with the many frozen entrees and frozen dinners that are now available in most supermarkets. Check labels for choices that contain about 300 calories, are less than 30 percent fat, contain at least 15 grams protein, and have less than 800 mg salt. There should be little or no sugar added, except possibly fructose.

Many frozen dinners and main dishes meet these criteria; however, many others do not. The following brands offer at least one frozen entree that can be fully recommended. (Because offerings and contents can change, we can't list specific dishes.)

Armour Dinner Classics Lite
Budget Gourmet [Slim Selects]
Dining Lites
Healthy Choice Meals
Le Menu Light Style Dinners
Stouffer's Lean Cuisine
Tyson Gourmet Selection
Weight Watchers

CHAPTER TEN

The G-Index Food Exchange Lists

The most effective and comprehensive approach to designing your own G-Index Diet is the food exchange concept. Simply stated, this technique involves eating each day a given number of exchanges (or servings, as I prefer to call them) from six major food groups.

Each food group or exchange list contains foods that are very similar in their content of carbohydrate, protein, fat, and calories. Thus, for most practical purposes, a serving size of any food within one food group—for example, a fruit—is nutritionally equivalent to, and may be substituted for, a specific amount of any other food in that group. The exchange lists that follow tell precisely how much of one food may substitute for another. For example, how many strawberries are nutritionally equivalent to a number of canned pears.

The nutritional exchange system was developed by the American Dietetics Association, the professional organization of registered dietitians, together with the American Diabetes Association. Its major advantage is that once you select the calorie level of your diet, you can forget the calorie or nutritional values of individual foods. These concerns have been taken care of by the nutritionists who designed the system. All you have to think about is the number of servings you should eat from each of the six food groups in the course of a day.

Well, not quite all. The food group exchange system developed before we understood the G-Index. Foods within each food group often have very different G-Indexes, even though their calorie, carbohydrate, protein, and fat content are similar. What we've done in this book is modify the food group exchange lists to take into account different foods' G-Index effect.

GETTING STARTED

Select your particular calorie level and then forget about calories and the nutritional balance of your meals. Most people who want to lose weight should go on the 1,200-calorie diet, though some very active men and women, or unusually large men, will be able to lose adequately on the 1,500-calorie regimen.

Most women find the 1,500-calorie program a good weight-maintenance level, and most men and athletic women do well holding their weight steady at 1,800 calories.

Athletic men and women may need extra calories to maintain their weight and meet their basic energy requirements. If you're in this category, you'll have to experiment by gradually adding extra servings—preferably from the fruit, vegetable, starch, or dairy groups—until your weight stabilizes.

The daily G-Index servings in the six major food groups are as follows:

Food Group	1,200 CAL	1,500 CAL	1,800 CAL
Milk/dairy	1.5	2.0	2.0
Vegetables	2	3	4
Fruit	4	4	4
Starch	5	6	8
Lean meat	5	6	6
Fat	1	2	4

These serving suggestions aren't rigid. There are some modifications you can make without violating the nutritional quality of your diet.

- You can eliminate one Starch serving each day and substitute one Fruit plus one Vegetable serving.
- You can eliminate one Milk/dairy serving each day and substitute one Fruit plus one Vegetable serving, *or* one Starch serving, *or* one medium Fat serving. (*Caution:* Decreasing your dairy foods usually requires adding a 300 mg of calcium supplement for every Milk/dairy exchange you eliminate. See your physician or dietitian for guidance.)
- You can eliminate one Fruit serving and substitute instead two Vegetable servings.

You can also exercise some flexibility in the way you eat these foods during a given day by choosing the time you take in each food. In other words, you may prefer to eat your fruits for breakfast and as an afternoon snack, or you may like to have a piece of fruit at each meal and snack.

In general, though, unless you have a special preference for a certain kind of food during a particular meal, it's best to spread out your intake of different types of foods as evenly as possible throughout the day. Here are some suggested distributions of the food group servings for the three levels of diets.

1,200-CALORIE PROGRAM

Food Group	Breakfast	Lunch	Dinner	Snack #1	Snack #2
Milk/dairy	0.5	0.5	0.5	—	—
Vegetables	—	1	1	—	—
Fruit	1	1	1	1	—
Starch	1	1	2	—	1
Lean meat	0 or 1	1 or 2	3	—	—
Fat	—	—	1	—	—

1,500-CALORIE PROGRAM

Food Group	Breakfast	Lunch	Dinner	Snack #1	Snack #2
Milk/dairy	1	0.5	0.5	—	—
Vegetables	—	1	2	—	—
Fruit	1	1	1	1	—
Starch	2	1	2	—	1
Lean meat	0 or 1	1 or 2	4	—	—
Fat	1	—	1	—	—

1,800-CALORIE PROGRAM

Food Group	Breakfast	Lunch	Dinner	Snack #1	Snack #2
Milk/dairy	1	0.5	0.5	—	—
Vegetables	—	2	2	—	—
Fruit	1	1	1	1	—
Starch	2	2	2	1	1
Lean meat	0 or 1	1 or 2	4	—	—
Fat	1	1	1	—	1

Now you're ready for the actual exchange tables. There are nine main tables.

Starch exchanges, including starches prepared with fat
Meat and meat substitute exchanges
Vegetable exchanges
Fruit exchanges
Milk/dairy exchanges (all skim or low-fat)
Fat exchanges
Free Food exchanges
Combination Food exchanges
Simple Sugar exchanges

The first six tables contain exchanges for the six major food groups; the last three—Free Food, Combination Food, and Simple Sugar—have been included to give you more flexibility in preparing your menus.

Before each table, I explain how the particular food group fits into the G-Index food exchange program. The tables show common foods in that group, the amount of the food that constitutes one serving, and its Glycemic Index classification.

Remember the ranking system: foods in categories 1 or 2 are desirable, those in category 3 are moderately desirable, and those in category 4 are less desirable. These rankings do *not* indicate the nutritional value; they simply show whether or not the food triggers hunger.

Also, with some fats or fat-containing foods, the GI ranking is ''1*.'' The asterisk reminds you that fats, when used properly, can suppress hunger. But their amounts must be *strictly limited*, or you will add unwanted pounds and may upset a healthy balance in your blood lipids, such as cholesterol.

STARCH EXCHANGES

Each serving contains approximately 15 grams of carbohydrate, 3 grams of protein, minimal fat, and 80 calories.

Starches are among the most favored foods in the American diet, and many starches have a favorable GI. But some popular starches are in class 3 or 4, so you'll have to closely watch the GI rankings in the right-hand column.

It's best to choose only Starch exchanges that are class 1 or 2. But many people can tolerate eating up to two of their Starch exchanges each day from among class 3 and 4 foods. Monitor your reactions to see if you can manage a few items that are higher on the Glycemic Index. If you can't, stick to those in the 1 or 2 slot.

STARCH FOODS—1 STARCH EXCHANGE

Food Item	Serving Size	G-Index

CEREALS, GRAINS, PASTA (See also cereal lists on pages 56–57 and 190.)

Breakfast Cereals

Cold Cereals

Food Item	Serving Size	G-Index
Most sweetened cold cereals— corn flakes, Muesli, Weetabix	½ cup	4
Most unsweetened cold cereals—shredded wheat	¾ cup	4
High-bran, spaghetti-shaped cereals—Fiber One, All-Bran with Extra Fiber	⅔ cup	2
Bran flakes	½ cup	4
Cereal with psyllium— Fiberwise	⅔ cup	2
Puffed cereals— Puffed rice	1.5 cup	4
Puffed Kashi	1 cup	4

Hot Cereals

Food Item	Serving Size	G-Index
Most processed, ready-to-eat, or precooked wheat or rice cereals—Wheatena, Cream of Rice	½ cup	4
Old-fashioned oatmeal	½ cup	⅔
Fine-grain oatmeal	½ cup	3
Instant oatmeal	½ cup	4
Oat bran	½ cup	3
Whole Kashi Breakfast Pilaf	¼ cup	2

Other Cereals, Grains, and Pasta

Food Item	Serving Size	G-Index
Barley	⅓ cup	1
Bulgur	½ cup (cooked)	2
Couscous	⅓ cup	2
Cornmeal	2½ tablespoons (raw)	3

Food Item	Serving Size	G-Index
Millet	¾ cup	4
Pasta (white or whole wheat)	½ cup (cooked)	2
Rice (white or brown)	⅓ cup (cooked)	3 or 4

COMMERCIAL BREADS (See also bread lists on pages 54 and 192.)

Standard white bread	1-ounce slice	4
Most commercial whole wheat breads	1-ounce slice	4
Diet wheat bread[1]	2 slices	4
100% stoneground whole wheat bread[2]—Vermont Bread Company, Brown Hills Organic Sesame, Brownberry Breads, Jewel Company Bread	1-ounce slice	3
100% sprouted or cracked wheat breads—		
Shiloh Farms	1-ounce slice	2
Alvarado Farms bagel	⅓	2
Commercial pumpernickel bread	1-ounce slice	3
Commercial rye bread (American-style)	1-ounce slice	4
100% whole-grain rye bread (coarse, European-style)—Braunschlagger	1-ounce slice	2
Pita (whole wheat or regular)	½ a 6-inch round 1 ounce	2

1. Most diet breads are digested quickly into sugar and are high on the G-Index. However, because diet breads have only half the calories of regular bread, use them in small amounts to *reduce* total bread calories.
2. Prefer coarse-textured brands. Most major brands offer a 100 percent stoneground whole wheat bread, but read the label carefully. Some breads called "stoneground" have bleached white flour as their largest component. Others have flour stoneground too fine. Check your local bakery and health food stores, as well as supermarkets.

Food Item	Serving Size	G-Index
Other Bread Products		
Bagel	½ small, 1 ounce	4
Breadsticks, crisp	2 (4 inch × ½ inch, ⅔ ounce)	4
Croutons, low-fat	1 cup	4
English muffin—Thomas's	½ muffin	4
Hot dog or hamburger bun	½ (1 ounce)	4
Plain roll, small	1 (1 ounce)	4
Raisin bread, unfrosted	1-ounce slice	4
BEANS, PEAS, LENTILS		
Most beans and peas, including kidney, butter beans, chickpeas[1]	⅓ cup (cooked)	1
Lentils	⅓ cup (cooked)	1
Baked beans	¼ cup	1
STARCHY VEGETABLES		
Corn kernels	½ cup	3
Corn-on-the-cob	1 6-inch ear	3
Lima beans	⅓ cup (cooked)	4
Peas, green (canned or frozen)	½ cup	1
Potato—		
baked	1 small (3 ounces)	4
boiled	1 small (3 ounces)	3
instant	3 ounces	4
mashed	½ cup	4
Squash, winter (acorn, butternut)[2]	¾ cup	3
Yam or sweet potato, plain	⅓ cup	2

CRACKERS, SNACKS (See also crackers, snacks, and muffins list, page 58.)

Animal Crackers	8	4

1. For lima beans, see starchy vegetables.
2. See Vegetable list for summer squash.

Food Item	Serving Size	G-Index
Creamsicle—sugar-free Cream Pops	3	2
Fig Newton	1½	2
R. W. Frookie (high-fructose cookie, fat free)*	2	2
R. W. Frookie Apple Fruiting cookie*	1⅓	2
R. W. Frookie Frookwich*	1½	2
Graham crackers	3 (2½-inch)	3
Health Valley*—		
Apple Fruit Bar	½	2
Apple Spice Muffin	⅔	2
Fat-Free Granola Bar	½	2
Fruit & Fitness Cookies	2	2
Matzoh, regular	¾ board (¾ ounce)	4
Matzoh, 100% stoneground whole wheat—Goodman's, Manischewitz	¾ board (¾ ounce)	2
Melba toast	5	4
Muffins—		
Apples 'n' Oats (GI recipe)	1	1
Muffin-a-Day[1]		
Carrot flavor	½	2
Apple-banana flavor	½	1

*Health food specialty brands such as R. W. Frookie, Health Valley, and Nature's Choice make many foods that are low in fat and have a low G-Index. However, they also make products that have a high G-Index. We have not been able to test more than a few of the many available "health foods," therefore you will often have to make a "best guess" about a food's G-Index by reading its label. If the label has whole grain and fructose listed as main ingredients then you know the contents have a low G-Index.

A "health" food is likely to have a moderately low G-Index if the first or second ingredient is a low G-Index fruit or fruit juice, or a whole grain, cracked, or sprouted grain. Ignore claims made on the wrapper that are not confirmed on the label. The G-Index is likely to be high if the first two ingredients are whole wheat but not whole grain, cracked, or sprouted wheat, and/or raisins, dates, pineapple, honey, or molasses.

1. These are low-fat muffins. Most other commercial muffins contain fat; see "Starch Foods Prepared with Fats." Mufin-A-Day can be ordered by telephone: 1-800-258-8961.

Food Item	Serving Size	G-Index
Nature's Choice Oat Bran Bars*	1	2
Nature's Warehouse Juice Flavored Pastry Popover	1	1
Oyster crackers	24	4
Popcorn, air-popped, no fat added	3 cups	4
Pretzels	¾ ounce	4
Rye crisp from processed flour	1-ounce slice	4
Rye crisp from 100% whole grain—		
Ry Krisp	4 triple	3
Wasa Crispbread	1½	3
Ryvita Crisp Bread	3	3
Crisp Bread	4	3
Kavli Crispbread	7	3
Saltines	6	4
Whole wheat crackers (no fat added)	2–4 slices (¾ ounce)	4
Frozen yogurt, nonfat— sugar-free, artificial sweetener		
added	4 ounces	2
sugar added	3 ounces	4
Frozen yogurt, regular		
sugar added	2.5 ounces	4
Ultra Slim-Fast French Vanilla Shake	4 ounces	2

STARCH FOODS PREPARED WITH FAT—
1 STARCH EXCHANGE + 1 FAT EXCHANGE

Food Item	Serving Size	G-Index (MF = Medium Fat Content)
Biscuit	1 (2-inch)	3
Chow mein noodles	½ cup	3
Corn bread	1 (2-inch square, 2 ounces)	3
Cracker, round butter type	6	3
French-fried potatoes	10 (2 to 3½-inch, 1.5 ounces)	3
Morning Snack AM Fiber Bar— strawberry or oatmeal and almond	½	1
Muffins Blueberry Oat Bran (GI recipe)	1 (2 ounces)	1
muffins, plain	1 (2 ounces)[1]	3
Pancakes	2 (4-inch)	3
Stuffing, prepared bread	¼ cup	3
Taco shells	2 (6-inch)	3
Waffle	1 (4½-inch square)	3
Whole wheat crackers, fat added, such as Triscuits	4–6 (1 ounce)	3
Fructose-sweetened Cookies— Fifty 50	3	2
R. W. Frookie	2	2

1. One rarely finds a 2-ounce commercial muffin these days. Most are 5 ounces or more— 8 ounces is not unusual. At about 125 calories per ounce, one large muffin could be an entire day's calorie intake.

MEAT EXCHANGES

Meats and meat substitutes such as cheese are the main sources of protein for most Americans. But meats are also our main source of high-calorie fat.

The following list is divided into lean, medium, and high-fat foods. To meet the taste demands of the majority of dieters, we've used medium-fat meats as the basis for our exchanges. But when possible, choose *lean* meats. You may then increase your meat portion by one-third, with no increase in calories. For example, instead of five medium-fat meat exchanges per day, you can have 6⅔ lean meat exchanges. High-fat meats should be eaten only rarely.

Note: It's possible to omit all true meat foods and still obtain all the protein you need from meat substitutes, such as milk products, or from vegetable foods, such as soybeans, peanuts, nuts, seeds, or careful combinations of grains and beans.

Here's a specific nutritional breakdown of the three types of meats:

NUTRITIONAL CONTENT OF ONE MEAT EXCHANGE

Type	Carbohydrate (g)	Protein (g)	Fat (g)	Calories
Lean	0	7	3	55
Medium fat (MF)	0	7	5	75
High fat (HF)	0	7	8	100

As you can see, there is no carbohydrate in meat. As I indicated earlier, the traditional, narrow definition of the Glycemic Index doesn't apply to meats. But since meat doesn't raise the blood sugar very much and in general operates like a low GI food, I've categorized all the following meats as a "1*." The asterisk, you'll recall, reminds us that meat isn't a true low GI food, but *acts* like a GI food.

A difficult issue with meats, however, is fat content. High fat will ruin any diet, including the G-Index Diet. On the other hand, menus that are too low in fat can endanger the mechanism that controls blood sugar and insulin. So one goal of our diet has been to place the right amount of fat (always a relatively small amount) at the right time during the day to help you maintain consumption of relatively low fat calories.

LEAN MEAT AND SUBSTITUTES—1 MEAT EXCHANGE (55 CALORIES)

Food Item	Serving Size (Weight After Cooking)[1]
Beef: USDA Good or Choice grades of lean cuts, such as round, sirloin, flank steak, tenderloin, or chipped beef (high salt)	1 ounce
Pork: lean cuts such as fresh ham; canned, cured, or boiled ham (high salt); Canadian bacon (high salt), tenderloin	1 ounce
Veal: all cuts except veal cutlets (ground or cubed)	1 ounce
Poultry: skinless chicken, turkey, Cornish hen	1 ounce
Fish—	
All fresh and frozen fish	1 ounce
Crab, lobster, scallops, shrimp, clams, fresh or canned in water (high salt)	2 ounces
Tuna, canned in water (high salt)	¼ cup (2 ounces)
Herring, uncreamed or smoked	1 ounce
Sardines, canned	2 medium
Game—	

1. As a rule of thumb, cooking shrinks meat weight by about 25%.

Food Item	Serving Size (Weight After Cooking)[1]
Venison, rabbit	1 ounce
Pheasant, duck, goose (without skin)	1 ounce
Cheese—	
Any cottage cheese	¼ cup
Grated Parmesan	2 tablespoons
Diet cheeses (with less than 55 calories/ounce—high salt)[2]	1 ounce
Other—	
95% fat-free luncheon meat	1 ounce
Egg whites	3
Egg substitutes with less than 55 calories/per ¼ cup	¼ cup

MEDIUM-FAT MEAT (MF) AND SUBSTITUTES—
1 MEAT EXCHANGE
(75 CALORIES)

Food Item	Serving Size (Weight After Cooking) (MF)
Beef: Most beef products—all ground beef, roast (rib, chuck, rump), steak (cube, porterhouse, T-bone), and meatloaf	1 ounce
Pork: Most pork products—chops, loin, roast, Boston butt, cutlets	1 ounce

1. As a rule of thumb, cooking shrinks meat weight by about 25%.
2. See also diet cheese list, page 190.

Food Item	Serving Size (Weight After Cooking) (MF)
Lamb: Most lamb products—chops, leg, roast	1 ounce
Veal: Cutlet, ground or cubed, unbreaded	1 ounce
Poultry: Chicken with skin, ground turkey, duck, or goose well drained of fat	1 ounce
Fish—	
Tuna, canned in oil and drained (high salt)	1 ounce
Salmon, canned (high salt)	1 ounce
Cheese: Skim or part-skim cheeses—mozzarella, ricotta, diet cheeses (with 56–80 calories per ounce)	1 ounce
Other—	
86% fat-free luncheon meat (high salt)	1 ounce
Egg (high in cholesterol—people with a cholesterol problem should limit to about 3 a week)	1
Tofu	4 ounces (2½ × 2¾ × 1 inch)
Liver, heart, kidney, sweetbreads (high in cholesterol)	1 ounce

HIGH-FAT MEAT AND SUBSTITUTES—
1 MEAT EXCHANGE
(100 CALORIES)*

Food Item	Amount for One High-fat Meat Exchange (Weight Given After Cooking) (HF)
Beef: Most USDA Prime cuts of beef—ribs, corned beef (high salt)	1 ounce
Pork: Spareribs, ground pork, pork sausage (high salt)	1 ounce
Lamb: Ground lamb	1 ounce
Fish: Any fried fish	1 ounce
Cheese: All regular cheeses (high salt)—American, blue, cheddar, Monterey Jack, Swiss	1 ounce
Other—	
Luncheon meat (high salt)—bologna, salami, pimiento loaf	1 ounce
Sausage (high salt)—Polish, Italian, Knockwurst	1 ounce
Bratwurst (high salt), frankfurter (chicken or turkey)	1 ounce
Peanut butter	1 tablespoon
Frankfurter—beef, pork, or combination (high salt)	1 (1.6 ounces)[1]

VEGETABLE EXCHANGES

With only a few exceptions, vegetables have a desirable class 1 Glycemic Index as well as low amounts of fat. They are

*Except for peanut butter and fried fish (depending on the oil it is fried in), these foods are all high in saturated fat, which should be strictly limited by people with a cholesterol problem.

1. Counts as one high-fat Meat exchange plus one Fat exchange.

also usually high in vitamins, minerals, and dietary fiber. One Vegetable exchange contains 5 grams of carbohydrate, 2 grams of protein, and 25 calories.

With few exceptions (such as carrots), vegetables contain little carbohydrate. So even though the potential GI of their carbohydrate would be high if large amounts were consumed, as a practical matter the GI effect of normal portions of these vegetables is negligible. Hence, vegetables, by and large, rate a solid class 1 on the G-Index.

Finally, many vegetables are so low in calories that they appear on the Free Food exchange lists, rather than on this Vegetable exchange list.

Note: All fresh and frozen unprocessed vegetables are very low in salt, but canned vegetables usually have salt added. Much of this salt can be removed by rinsing the vegetables after removing them from the can.

Here are a few practical guidelines as you prepare to use the vegetable list:

- For all raw vegetables, one Vegetable exchange equals 1 cup of raw vegetables.
- For all cooked vegetables, one Vegetable exchange equals ½ cup of cooked vegetables.
- For all vegetable juices, one Vegetable exchange equals ½ cup juice.

But here are some exceptions:

- For artichokes, one Vegetable exchange equals ½ medium artichoke.
- For tomatoes, one Vegetable exchange equals one large tomato.

VEGETABLES—1 VEGETABLE EXCHANGE

Food Item	G-Index
Artichoke	1
Asparagus	1
Beans (green, wax, Italian)	1
Bean sprouts	1
Beets	3
Broccoli	1
Brussels sprouts	1
Cabbage, cooked	1
Carrots [1]	4
Cauliflower	1
Greens (collard, mustard, turnip)	1
Kohlrabi	1
Leeks	1
Mushrooms, cooked	1
Okra	1
Onions	1
Peppers (green)	1
Rutabaga	1
Sauerkraut (high salt)	1
Snow Peas	2
Spinach, cooked	1
Squash, summer (see Starch list for winter squash)	1
Tomato	1
Tomato/vegetable juice	1
Carrot juice	4
Turnips	4
Water chestnuts	1
Zucchini (cooked)	1

1. Even though ounce-for-ounce carrots and carrot juice trigger a greater rise in blood sugar than other vegetables, they may still be eaten in moderation. Modest amounts are tolerated because one Vegetable exchange is a very small portion (only 25 calories). For example, one Vegetable exchange contains much fewer carbohydrate calories than does a Starch exchange or a Fruit exchange. Thus, one medium carrot—about one Vegetable exchange—provides only one-third the carbohydrate calories of a slice of bread. Eating one carrot (G-Index 4) has only a modest effect on blood sugar; however, eating two, three, or four carrots causes a dramatic rise in blood sugar.

FRUIT EXCHANGES

The fruits may be fresh, frozen, or canned *without* added sugar.

One fruit exchange contains approximately 15 grams of carbohydrate, no protein or fat, and 60 calories. With only a few exceptions—such as dried fruits like raisins and dates—fruits rank well on the Glycemic Index.

Fruit juices are also class 1 foods on the G-Index, but because they are liquid and require no chewing, it's easy to take in more than you intend. In contrast, whole fruit requires more work and also contains more fiber. Therefore, whole fruit is preferable to juice.

FRUIT—1 FRUIT EXCHANGE

Food Item	Serving Size	G-Index
DRIED, FRESH, FROZEN, AND UNSWEETENED CANNED FRUIT		
Apple, fresh	1 (2-inch)	1
Applesauce, unsweetened	½ cup	1
Apricots, fresh	4 medium	1
Apricots, canned	4 halves	1
Banana	½ (9-inch)	2 or 3
Blackberries, fresh	¾ cup	1
Blueberries, fresh	¾ cup	1
Cantaloupe	⅓ (5-inch)	1
Cantaloupe, cubed	1 cup	1
Cherries, fresh	12 large	1
Cherries, canned	½ cup	1
Grapefruit, fresh	½ medium	1
Grapefruit, segments	¾ cup	1
Grapes	15 small	1
Honeydew melon	⅛ medium	1
Honeydew, cubed	1 cup	1
Kiwi	1 large	3
Mango	½	2
Nectarine	1 medium	1
Orange	1 small	1

Food Item	Serving Size	G-Index
Papaya, cubed	1 cup	1
Peach, fresh	1 (2¾ inches) or ¾ cup	1
Peach, canned	½ cup or 2 halves	1
Pear, fresh	½ large or 1 small	1
Pear, canned	½ cup or 2 halves	1
Persimmon	2 medium	1
Pineapple, fresh cubed	¾ cup	3 or 4
Plum, fresh	2 (2 inch)	1
Pomegranate	½	1
Raspberries, fresh	1 cup	1
Raisins	2 tablespoons	3 or 4
Strawberries, fresh	1¼ cups	1
Tangerine	2 (2½ inches)	1
Watermelon, cubed	1¼ cups	4

FRUIT JUICE (UNSWEETENED ONLY)

Apple juice or cider	½ cup	1
Cranberry [1]	⅓ cup	1
Grapefruit	½ cup	1
Grape	⅓ cup	1
Orange	½ cup	1
Pineapple	½ cup	3 or 4

MILK/DAIRY EXCHANGES

Milk products are an excellent source of protein and calcium, and the Glycemic Index of milk sugar (lactose) is very favorable.

The calorie value of one Milk dairy exchange varies depending on its fat content. The G-Index Diet assumes that,

---

1. Most commercial cranberry juices (other than diet versions) have substantial corn syrup or other high G-Index sweeteners added.

for the most part, you'll use skim or *very* low-fat (1 percent) milk products.

The milk category next highest in fat is called low-fat by professional dietitians. But at 5 grams of fat per exchange, one of these low-fat Milk/dairy exchanges contains as much fat as one medium-fat Meat exchange or one Fat exchange.

To help you keep these choices in perspective, I've labeled the traditional low-fat milk products as medium fat (MF) in the exchanges. Similarly, the highest fat Milk/dairy exchange is usually labeled whole milk by dietitians. I do *not* recommend this for people on the G-Index Diet. But if you should occasionally find yourself having to use whole milk, as sometimes happens when you're eating breakfast in a restaurant, think of it as a high fat food on our exchanges (HF).

An excellent way to sweeten a Milk/dairy serving, especially plain yogurt, is to combine it with one Fruit exchange, either mixed into the yogurt or eaten on the side.

A note on yogurt, cottage cheese, other cheeses, and ice cream. The recent availability of excellent-tasting, nonfat and low-fat frozen yogurt provides an attractive dessert or snack opportunity for the G-Index dieter. Nonfat yogurt usually contains 20 calories per ounce, and the low-fat variety has 30 calories.

Cottage cheese can be used to satisfy either the Meat or Milk/dairy requirement. Because of their relatively high fat content, many cheeses are considered moderate or high-fat Meat substitutes instead of Milk/dairy products. Ice cream—a very high fat food—is not considered a ''Milk'' under The Exchange List systems. Butter is listed under Fats.

More on lactose intolerance. A significant percentage of Americans have difficulty digesting milk sugar or lactose. This condition is known as lactose intolerance. Milk and ice cream often cause diarrhea or severe intestinal gas. But many people who cannot drink regular milk may still be comfortable with moderate amounts of buttermilk, yogurt, or cheese, since these foods contain less lactose.

Another solution is to take lactase digestive enzymes, which help you digest lactose; they can be put into or taken with milk products. Usually, but not always, these supplements prevent or reduce symptoms of lactose intolerance. Lactase is available without a prescription at most drug stores and health food stores.

A true milk allergy is much less frequent than lactose digestive deficiency. People with a true milk allergy should avoid all products with milk protein.

As you use the following dairy exchanges, you should be aware that Milk/dairy exchange contains the following components:

Type	Carbohydrates	Protein	Fat	Calories
Skim or very low-fat milk products (0–1% fat)	12	8	trace	90
Moderate-fat milk products (2% fat)	12	8	5	120 (MF)
Whole milk products (3.25% or more fat)	12	8	8	150 (HF)

SKIM MILK PRODUCTS—1 MILK/DAIRY EXCHANGE

Food Item	Serving Size	G-Index
Skim milk	1 cup	1
1 percent milk	1 cup	1
Buttermilk	1 cup	1
Evaporated skim milk	½ cup	1
Nonfat dry milk	⅓ cup	1
Yogurt—		
Plain nonfat	8 ounces	1
Nonfat, fruited, sugar-free (artificial sweetener added)	7 ounces	1
Nonfat, fruited, sugar added	5 ounces	4

Food Item	Serving Size	G-Index
Yogurt, frozen—[1]		
Honey Hills Farm nonfat, sugar-free	4.5 ounces	2
I Can't Believe It's Yogurt Yoglace	8 ounces	1
Baskin-Robbins nonfat strawberry, sugar-free	4 ounces	2

MODERATE-FAT MILK PRODUCTS— 1 MILK/DAIRY EXCHANGE

Food Item	Serving Size	G-Index (MF)
2% milk	1 cup	1
Plain low-fat yogurt (with added nonfat milk solids)	8 ounces	1
Low-fat yogurt with added natural sweetener	8 ounces	1
"Low-fat" frozen yogurt (30 calories per ounce with added natural sweetener)	4 ounces	1

1. For most brands of frozen yogurts, see Starch exchange, Crackers, Snacks. We are aware of only these three brands of frozen yogurt that have enough protein to qualify for the Milk and dairy exchange list.

WHOLE-MILK PRODUCTS—
1 MILK/DAIRY EXCHANGE*

Food Item	Serving Size	G-Index (HF)
Whole milk	1 cup	1
Evaporated whole milk	½ cup	1
Whole plain yogurt	8 ounces	1

FAT EXCHANGES

All fats are high in calories. Nuts, peanuts, and seeds contain substantial protein as well, and could be classified as meat substitutes. But unless you are planning a strictly vegetarian food day, the fat content of these foods is too high to routinely use to obtain your protein.

Because of their high-caloric content, fat foods should be taken in modest amounts and measured carefully. Saturated-fat foods should be especially limited by people with a cholesterol problem.

Still, everyone needs a specific minimum of fat in the diet. As fat intake gets very low, the appetite-enhancing effect of high Glycemic Index foods becomes more pronounced. Also, a small amount of fat is required for the body's healthy metabolic function. This is particularly true of unsaturated fats, which are found most abundantly in vegetables and fish.

Foods containing one Fat exchange have been flagged as moderate fat (MF). Depending on the caloric content of the product, you can eat more of certain fat foods than others while still getting one exchange of Fat amounting to 45 calories. For example, one teaspoon of margarine and one table-

* We do not recommend using whole-milk dairy products except in unusual situations. Foods from this list are noted in the food plan menus as (HF) for high fat.

spoon (3 teaspoons) of diet margarine have equivalent fat contents.

A note on fats and the Glycemic Index. As you now know, by scientific definition the Glycemic Index applies only to carbohydrates. Fat foods like meats contain little carbohydrate. Strictly speaking, these foods have no Glycemic Index. But to help you choose foods that won't disrupt blood sugar, I've stretched the concept to cover fats. This way, *all* foods that keep blood sugar levels steady receive a highly favorable 1 rating.

But fats cannot be eaten in limitless amounts. Quite the contrary, fat servings are strictly limited on this diet. A relatively low-fat diet is essential for weight control as well as for good health.

MAINLY UNSATURATED FATS—1 FAT EXCHANGE

Food Item	Serving Size	G-Index (MF)
Avocado	⅛ medium	1
Margarine	1 teaspoon	1
Diet margarine	1 tablespoon	1
Mayonnaise	1 teaspoon	1
Mayonnaise, reduced-calorie	1 tablespoon	1
NUTS AND SEEDS		
almond, dry-roasted	6 whole	1
cashews, dry-roasted	1 tablespoon	1
pecans	2 whole	1
peanuts	20 small or 10 large	1
walnuts	2 whole	1
other nuts	1 tablespoon	1
Seeds, pignoli, sunflower, without shells (beware, if salt added)	1 tablespoon	1
Pumpkin seeds	2 tablespoons	1

Food Item	Serving Size	G-Index (MF)
Vegetable oils (corn, cottonseed, safflower, soybean, sunflower, olive, peanut)	1 teaspoon	1
Olives (moderate salt)	10 small or 5 large	1
Salad dressing—		
Mayonnaise-type	1 tablespoon	1
Standard varieties	1 tablespoon	1
Reduced-calorie (20 calories)[1]	2 tablespoons	
Nonfat (varies from 2–16 calories per teaspoon	—	1

MAINLY SATURATED FATS—1 FAT EXCHANGE

Food Item	Serving Size	G-Index (HF)
Butter	1 teaspoon	1
Bacon (moderate salt)	1 slice	1
Chitterlings	½ ounce	1
Coconut, shredded	2 tablespoons	1
Coffee creamer, liquid	2 tablespoons	1
Coffee creamer, powder	4 teaspoons	1
Cream (light, coffee, table)	2 tablespoons	1
Cream, sour	2 tablespoons	1
Cream, heavy whipping	1 tablespoon	1
Cream cheese, regular	1½ tablespoons	1
Cream cheese, light	1 tablespoon	1
Nondairy low-fat whipped topping	3 tablespoons	1
Imitation sour cream	2 tablespoons	1

1. The first 2 tablespoons per ounce of low-calorie salad dressing is considered a free food.

FREE FOOD EXCHANGES

Foods that contain fewer than 20 calories per serving have minimal impact on weight, blood sugar, and fat metabolism. Therefore, they may be considered free foods.

The foods in this list that have specific serving sizes indicated may be eaten two or three times a day. Other free foods, which have no indication of portion sizes, may be eaten more or less as you wish—but they should be spread out over the entire day.

All of these foods are class 1 on the G-Index.

FREE FOOD EXCHANGES

DRINKS

Bouillon (high salt and salt-free varieties)
Broth without fat
Carbonated drinks, sugar-free
Carbonated water, club soda, or seltzer
Cocoa powder, unsweetened (1 tablespoon) (For example, add to milk serving with non-calorie sweetener.)
Coffee/Tea, caffeine-free [1]
Drink mixes, sugar-free
Tonic water, sugar-free

VEGETABLES (raw, 1 cup)

Cabbage
Celery

---

1. Caffeine promotes blood sugar instability. Although caffeinated coffee and tea are free foods from a calorie perspective, their Glycemic Index is class 4. See page 76 for a discussion of caffeine.

Chinese cabbage
Cucumber
Green onions
Hot peppers
Mushrooms
Radishes
Zucchini

SALAD GREENS

Endive
Escarole
Lettuce
Romaine
Spinach

SWEET SUBSTITUTES

Gelatin, sugar-free
Gum, sugar-free
Hard candy, sugar-free
Jam or Jelly, sugar-free (2 teaspoons)
Pancake syrup, sugar-free (1–2 tablespoons)
Sugar substitutes—aspartame, saccharin
Very low calorie whipped toppings (2 tablespoons)

CONDIMENTS

Catsup (1 tablespoon)
Horseradish
Mustard
Pickles, dill, unsweetened (high salt)
Salad dressing, very low calorie—no more than 10 calories/
   tablespoon variety (2 tablespoons)

SEASONINGS[1]

Basil
Celery seeds

---

1. Seasonings help enliven the taste of many foods. Limit those that contain sodium or salt.

Cinnamon
Chili powder
Chives
Curry
Dill
Flavoring extracts—i.e., vanilla, almond, walnut, peppermint,
  butter, lemon
Garlic
Garlic powder
Herbs
Hot pepper sauce
Lemon
Lemon juice
Lime
Lime juice
Mint
Onion powder
Oregano
Paprika
Pepper
Pimiento
Spices
Soy sauce, regular (high salt)
Soy sauce, low-sodium (tahini)
Wine, used in cooking (¼ cup)
Worcestershire sauce

COMBINATION FOODS EXCHANGES

Many common foods contain combinations of products, that
overlap exchange lists. When you eat these, credit them to
each relevant exchange category.

COMBINATION FOODS

Food Item	Serving Size	Exchange Equivalent	G-Index
Casseroles	1 cup (8 ounces)	2 Starch 2 medium-fat Meat 1 Fat	2 (HF)
Cheese pizza, thin crust (high salt) ¼ of a 10-inch or 15-ounce pizza	2 Starch 1 medium-fat Meat 1 Fat	2 (HF)	
Chili with beans, commercial (high salt)	1 cup (8 ounces)	2 Starch 2 medium-fat Meat 2 Fat	1 (HF)
Chow mein (high salt)	2 cups (16 ounces)	1 Starch 2 Vegetable 2 lean Meat	2
Macaroni and cheese	1 cup (8 ounces)	2 Starch 1 medium-fat Meat 2 Fat	1 (HF)

SOUPS, LOW-FAT—

Campbell's Healthy Request			
Hearty Chicken Noodle	8 ounces	1 Starch	2
Hearty Minestrone	8 ounces	1 Starch	2
Tomato (contains corn syrup)	8 ounces	1 Starch	3
Health Valley			
Mushroom Barley	6 ounces	1 Starch	1
Tomato	5 ounces	1 Starch	1

Food Item	Serving Size	Exchange Equivalent	G-Index
Lipton's Cup-a-Soup, Chicken Noodle (contains corn syrup)	8 ounces	1 Starch	3
Nile Spice			
Couscous Vegetable	5 ounces	1 Starch	1
Chicken Soup with almonds	5 ounces	1 Starch	1
Couscous Lentil Curry Soup	5 ounces	1 Starch	1
Pritikin			
Vegetable Soup	8 ounces	1 Starch	1
Progresso			
Vegetable	10.5 ounces	1 Starch	1

GENERIC COMMERCIAL SOUPS [1]

Food Item	Serving Size	Exchange Equivalent	G-Index
Bean (high salt)	1 cup (8 ounces)	1 Starch 1 Vegetable 1 lean Meat	1
Chunky, all varieties (high salt)	10¾ ounces	1 Starch 1 Vegetable 1 medium-fat Meat	(MF)

1. Many—but far from all—supermarket and health food store soups are low fat and low G-Index; they are tasty and make excellent choices for the G-Index diet. Exceptions from the many include creamed soups like New England clam chowder, soups with meat, and those with corn syrup or other sweeteners added. Be aware that most supermarket brands have considerable salt added; many from health stores do not. Recently, lower salt versions of supermarket soups have become widely available. Homemade soups do not necessarily require salt.

Food Item	Serving Size	Exchange Equivalent	G-Index
Cream, made with water (high salt)	1 cup (8 ounces)	1 Starch 1 Fat	1 (MF)
Vegetable (high salt)	1 cup (8 ounces)	1 Starch	2
Broth (high salt)	1 cup (8 ounces)	1 Starch	2

OTHER DISHES

Spaghetti and meatballs, canned (high salt)	1 cup (8 ounces)	2 Starch 1 medium-fat Meat 2 Fat	2 (HF)
Sugar-free pudding made with skim milk	½ cup	1 Starch	2

SIMPLE SUGAR EXCHANGES

Simple sugars contain about 15 calories per teaspoon. They are 100 percent carbohydrate and are poor in vitamins and minerals.

There is no nutritional need to eat simple sugars, but they may be used in moderation as a sweetener. Only one or two teaspoons should be consumed at a meal.

Unfortunately, large amounts of sugar can also be "hidden" in foods, so it's important to read your labels closely to see how much sugar you're taking in.

The Glycemic Index of simple sugars varies considerably. Class 1 sweeteners are obviously to be preferred; these include fructose, lactose, and artificial sweeteners. Sucrose, though only moderately desirable at class 3, can also be used sparingly.

SIMPLE SUGARS

Food Item	Approx. Calories per teaspoon	G-Index
Sucrose (table sugar)	15	3
Fructose (fruit sugar)	15	1
Honey	15	4
Lactose (milk sugar)	15	1
Molasses	15	4
Corn syrup	15	4
"High fructose" corn syrup	15	4
Jams and jellies (all fruit)	15–20	1
Jams and jellies with fructose added[1]	4–20	1
Jams and jellies with sucrose added	15–20	2
Jams and jellies, sugar-free	2	1

1. Calorie content varies widely. For example, Featherweight strawberry fruit spread with fructose contains only 4 calories per teaspoon.

CHAPTER ELEVEN

It's Not *Really* a Diet After All!

As you've probably discovered by now, the G-Index Diet isn't a diet in the traditional sense. To be sure, weight control is a primary goal. But this approach has some distinctive features that sets it apart from other weight-loss programs:

- The G-Index Diet is the missing element that now enables anyone to take weight off and keep it off *permanently*.
- Instead of focusing on calories, there is emphasis on nutritious foods that *suppress hunger*—items low on the Glycemic Index.
- There are no "forbidden foods." You can eat anything, so long as you abide by the basic ground rules of the program.
- Calories, fat, and other nutritional needs have been calculated for you and plugged into the basic diet plans.

In many ways, then, the G-Index approach is more a way of life than just another diet. Once you have learned to think in terms of low GI foods, you'll never again have to worry about depriving yourself or relying on your willpower to fight off hunger pangs.

As you may have noticed, the information in this book has

been presented as a series of building blocks that form the structure for you to move ever closer to freedom, independence, and satisfaction in your eating habits. First, you learned the basic scientific concepts behind the diet. Next, you saw how people with different types of weight problems have succeeded on it. Then, you found out how specific food products can trigger hunger or suppress it.

After establishing this foundation, you were provided a set of fixed menus and recipes, which took you step-by-step through a comprehensive, nutritionist-designed G-Index eating plan.

Next, you saw ways that you could branch out in your eating, beyond the given menus and recipes. Specifically, you were presented with tactics and suggestions that allow you to exercise flexibility yet remain consistent with the G-Index principles—whether at home or at a restaurant.

Finally, you've been provided with comprehensive food exchange lists that empower you to build your own menus and recipes. This is the final step that gives you the freedom to eat as you like, yet protects you from hunger pangs.

As you've moved through this process, you've seen that it's not necessary to count calories or fat grams. You've only had to learn which of your favorite foods are lowest on the Glycemic Index and then make them a prominent part of your daily fare.

If you're like me, you now have several favorite fruits, vegetables, dairy foods, and other products in mind that are low on the G-Index. You've probably arranged to make most, if not all, of them easily accessible, both at home and in your office. When hunger strikes, you now have the perfect weapons at hand: low GI foods that provide all the benefits of other low-fat diets *and also* keep you satisfied until the next meal.

You can see why the G-Index program is not just another diet. By any definition, this approach to eating can be a life-transforming experience for people who want to take weight off and keep it off forever. It has been for me, and I trust it will be for you as well.

BIBLIOGRAPHY

These references are scientific and technical. They will be useful mainly for health or nutrition professionals interested in the scientific basis of the G-Index diet and understanding related aspects of overweight problems.

American Diabetes Association. "Nutritional Recommendations and Principles for Individuals with Diabetes Mellitus." *Diabetes Care* 14 (1991): 20–26.

Anderson, J., L. Story, N. Zettwoch. "Metabolic Effects of Fructose Supplementation in Diabetic Individuals." *Diabetes Care* 12 (1989): 337–43.

Bellisle, F., F. Louis-Sylvestre, D. Demozay, et al. "Reflex Insulin Response Associated to Food Intake in Human Subjects." *Physiology and Behavior* 31 (1983): 515–21.

Brand, J., P. Nicholson, A. Thoburn, et al. "Food Processing and the Glycemic Index." *American Journal of Clinical Nutrition* 42 (1985): 1192–96.

Brand, J. "Glyceamic Index of Tropical Fruit and Australian Biscuits." *Proceedings of Nutrition of Australia* 15 (1990): 251.

Brand, J., B. J. Snow, G. Nabhan, et al. "Plasma Glucose and Insulin Responses to Traditional Pima Indian Meals." *American Journal of Clinical Nutrition* 51 (1990): 416–20.

Brand, J., K. Foster, S. Crossman, et al. "The Glycaemic and Insulin Indices of Realistic Meals and Rye Bread Tested in Health Subjects." *Diabetes, Nutrition and Metabolism* 3 (1990): 137–42.

Brand, J., S. Colagiuri, S. Crossman. "Low-Glycemic Index Foods Improve Long-Term Glycemic Control in NIDDM." *Diabetes Care* 14 (1991): 95–101.

Bray, G. "The Treatment for Obesity: A Nutrient Balance/ Nutrient Partition Approach." *Nutrition Reviews* 49 (1991): 33–44.

Bukar, J., N. Mezitis, V. Saitas, F. X. Pi-Sunyer. "Frozen Desserts and Glycemic Response in Well-controlled NIDDM Patients." *Diabetes Care* 13 (1990): 382–85.

Chew, I., J. Brand, A. Thoburn, et al. "Application of Glycemic Index to Mixed Meals." *American Journal of Clinical Nutrition* 47 (1988): 53–62.

Collier, G., T. Wolever, G. Wong. "Prediction of Glycemic Response to Mixed Meals in Noninsulin-Dependent Diabetic Subjects." *American Journal of Clinical Nutrition* 44 (1986): 349–52.

Cornell, C., J. Rodin, H. Weingarten. "Stimulus-Induced Eating When Satiated." *Physiology & Behavior* 45 (1989): 695–704.

Crapo, P., J. Scarlett, O. Kolterman. "Comparison of the Metabolic Responses to Fructose and Sucrose Sweetened Foods." *American Journal of Clinical Nutrition* 36 (1982): 256–61.

Friedman, M., I. Ramirez. "Relationship of Fat Metabolism to Food Intake." *American Journal of Clinical Nutrition* 42 (1985): 1093–98.

Guilliford, M., E. J. Bicknell, J. Scarpello, "Differential

Effect of Protein and Fat Ingestion on Blood Glucose Responses to High-and Low-Glycemic-Index Carbohydrates in Noninsulin-Dependent Diabetic Subjects." *American Journal of Clinical Nutrition* 50 1989: 773–77.

Hermansen, K., O. Rasmussen, J. Anfred, et al. "Glycemic Effects of Spaghetti and Potato Consumed as Part of Mixed Meal on NIDDM Patients." *Diabetes Care* 10 (1987): 401–5.

Jenkins, D., T. Wolever, A. Jenkins, et al. "The Glycemic Response to Carbohydrate Foods." *The Lancet*, August 18, 1984; pp. 388–91.

Jenkins, D., T. Wolever, J. Kalmusky. "Low Glycemic Index Carbohydrate Foods in the Management of Hyperlipidemia." *American Journal of Clinical Nutrition* 42 (1985): 604–17.

Jenkins, D., T. Wolever, G. Collier. "Metabolic Effects of a Low-Glycemic-Index Diet." *American Journal of Clinical Nutrition* 46 (1987): 968–75

Jenkins, D., T. Wolever, G. Buckley. "Low-Glycemic-Index Starchy Foods in the Diabetic Diet." *American Journal of Clinical Nutrition* 48 (1988): 248–54.

Karny I., C. Nernberg, Z. Madar. "Glycemic and Insulinemic Responses after Ingestion of Ethnic Foods by NIDDM and Healthy Subjects." *American Journal of Clinical Nutrition* 55 (1992): 89–95.

Levine, A., J. Tallman, M. Grace, et al. "Effect of Breakfast Cereals on Short-Term Food Intake." *American Journal of Clinical Nutrition* 50 (1989): 1303–7.

Mani, U., S. Bhatt, M. Nivedita. "Glycemic Index of Traditional Indian Carbohydrate Foods." *Journal of the American College of Nutrition* 9 (1990): 573–77.

Modan, M., H. Halkin. "Hyperinsulinemia or Increased Sympathetic Drive as Links for Obesity and Hypertension." *Diabetes Care* 14 (1991): 470–81.

Nielsen, P., G. Nielsen. "Preprandial Blood Glucose Values: Influences on Glycemic Response Studies." *American Journal of Clinical Nutrition* 49 (1989): 1243–46.

Nutrition Reviews. "The Metabolic Basis for the 'Apple' and the 'Pear' Body Habitus." *Nutrition Reviews* 49 (1991): 84–87.

Ritz, P., M. Krempf, D. Coarec. "Comparative Continuous-Indirect-Calorimetry Study of Two Carbohydrates with Different Glycemic Indices." *American Journal of Clinical Nutrition* 54 (1991): 855–59.

Rodin, J. "Insulin Levels, Hunger, and Food Intake: An Example of Feedback Loops in Body Weight Regulation." *Health Psychology* 4 (1985): 1–24.

Rodin, J., J. Wack, E. Ferrannini, et al. "Effect of Insulin and Glucose on Feeding Behavior." *Metabolism* 34 (1985): 826–31.

Rodin, J., D. Reed, L. Jamner. "Metabolic Effects of Fructose and Glucose: Implications for Food Intake." *American Journal of Clinical Nutrition* 47 (1988): 683–89.

Rolls, B. "Experimental Analyses of the Effects of Variety in a Meal on Human Feeding." *American Journal of Clinical Nutrition* 42 (1985): 932–39.

Rowe, J., J. Young, K. Minaker. "Effect of Insulin and Glucose Infusions on Sympathetic Nervous System Activity in Normal Man." *Diabetes* 30 (1981): 219–25.

Sahakian, B., M. Lean. "Salivation and Insulin Secretion in Response to Food in Non-obese Men and Women." *Appetite, Journal for Intake Research* 2 (1981): 209–16.

Schwarz, M., Y. Schutz, F. Foridevaux. "Thermogenesis in Men and Women Induced by Fructose vs. Glucose Added to a Meal." *American Journal of Clinical Nutrition* 49 (1989): 667–74.

Sheppard, L., A. Kristal, L. Kushi. "Weight Loss in Women

Participating in a Randomized Trial of Low-Fat Diets." *American Journal of Clinical Nutrition* 54 (1991): 821–28.

Simon, C., J. Schleinger, R. Sapin, et al. "Cephalic Phase Insulin Secretion in Relation to Food Presentation in Normal and Overweight Subjects." *Physiology & Behavior* 36 (1986): 465–69.

Thomas, D., J. Brotherhood, J. Brand. "Influence of Glycemic Index of the Pre-game Meal on Carbohydrate Metabolism." *Medicine and Science in Sports and Exercise* 22 (1990) (suppl., April): S 121.

Wardle, J., and H. Beinart. "Binge Eating: A Theoretical Review." *British Journal of Clinical Psychology* 20 (1981): 97–109.

Wolever, T., D. Jenkins, J. Kalmusky. "Glycemic Response to Pasta: Effect of Surface Area, Degree of Cooking and Protein Enrichment." *Diabetes Care* 9 (1986): 401–4.

Wolever, T., J. Jenkins, "The Use of the Glycemic Index in Predicting the Blood Glucose Response to Mixed Meals." *American Journal of Clinical Nutrition* 43 (1986): 167–72.

Wolever, T., D. Jenkins, A. Ocana. "Second-meal Effect: Low-Glycemic-Index Foods Eaten at Dinner Improve Subsequent Breakfast Glycemic Response." *American Journal of Clinical Nutrition* 48 (1988): 1041–47.

Wolever, T., A. Csima, D. Jenkins. "The Glycemic Index: Variation Between Subjects and Predictive Difference." *Journal of the American College of Nutrition* 8 (1989): 235–47.

Wolever, T. "Relationship Between Dietary Fiber Content and Composition in Foods and the Glycemic Index." *American Journal of Clinical Nutrition* 51 (1990): 72–75.

Wolever, T. "Metabolic Effects of Continuous Feeding." *Metabolism* 39 (1990): 947–51.

Wolever, T. "The Glycemic Index: Methodology and Clinical Implications." *American Journal of Clinical Nutrition* 54 (1991): 846–54.

Wolever, T., D. Jenkins, V. Vuksan, et al. "Glycemic Index of Foods in Individual Subjects." *Diabetes Care* 13 (1990): 126–32.

Wolever, T., V. Vuksan, H. Eshuis. "Effect of Method of Administration of Psyllium on Glycaemic Response and Carbohydrate Digestibility." *Journal of the American College of Nutrition* 10 (1991): 364–71.

Woods, S., D. Porte, E. Bobbioni. "Insulin: Its Relationship to the Central Nervous System and to the Control of Food Intake and Body Weight." *American Journal of Clinical Nutrition* 42 (1985): 1063–71

Zavaronia, I., E. Bonora, M. Pagliara, et al. "Risk Factors for Coronary Artery Disease in Health Persons with Hyperinsulinemia and Normal Glucose Tolerance." *New England Journal of Medicine* 320 (1989): 702–6.

INDEX

Boldface entries indicate recipes.